THRIVING
BEYOND
FIFTY

Also by Will Harlow

The 7 Steps to Overcome Sciatica (2018)

THRIVING
BEYOND
FIFTY

111 Natural Strategies to Restore Your Mobility,

Avoid Surgery and Stay Off Pain Pills for Good

Will Harlow MSc, MCSP, Cert. MA
Founder of the @HT-Physio YouTube channel

HAY HOUSE
Carlsbad, California • New York City
London • Sydney • New Delhi

Published in the United Kingdom by:
Hay House UK Ltd, The Sixth Floor, Watson House,
54 Baker Street, London W1U 7BU
Tel: +44 (0)20 3927 7290; www.hayhouse.co.uk

Published in the United States of America by:
Hay House LLC, PO Box 5100, Carlsbad, CA 92018-5100
Tel: (1) 760 431 7695 or (800) 654 5126; www.hayhouse.com

Published in Australia by:
Hay House Australia Publishing Pty Ltd, 18/36 Ralph St, Alexandria NSW 2015
Tel: (61) 2 9669 4299; www.hayhouse.com.au

Published in India by:
Hay House Publishers (India) Pvt Ltd, Muskaan Complex,
Plot No.3, B-2, Vasant Kunj, New Delhi 110 070
Tel: (91) 11 4176 1620; www.hayhouse.co.in

Text © Will Harlow, 2024

Photography © David Cummings, 2024

Cover art direction: Leanne Siu Anastasi
Cover design: Bryony Harlow and Vanessa Mendozzi

The moral rights of the author have been asserted.

A catalogue record for this book is available from the British Library.

Tradepaper ISBN: 978-1-4019-9418-1
E-book ISBN: 978-1-83782-419-9
Audiobook ISBN: 978-1-83782-417-5

Interior line illustrations: Shutterstock

10 9 8 7 6 5 4 3 2 1

Printed in the United States of America

This product uses responsibly sourced papers and/or recycled materials. For more information, see www.hayhouse.com.

To Mum and Dad, who encouraged my reading and
writing ever since I could hold a pencil.

To my grandparents, who are an endless source of inspiration
(I hope you find something useful in these pages).

And to B, for showing me nothing but support,
even during my early morning rituals.

"Don't let aging get you down. It's too hard to get back up."

JOHN WAGNER, COMIC BOOK AUTHOR

Contents

Part Five: Hips and Knees

Part Six: Feet and Ankles

Part Seven: Whole-Body Health

Part Eight: The Power of the Mind

List of Exercises

Why Did I Update
Thriving Beyond Fifty?

When I first wrote *Thriving Beyond Fifty*, I never imagined the impact that it would have. Published in 2020, the first edition went on to become a bestseller in two separate categories on Amazon, selling tens of thousands of copies worldwide in its first three years of publication. Initially dreamed up as not much more than a method of establishing credibility with potential clients for my physio (or, as it is also called: physical therapy) business, *Thriving Beyond Fifty* went on to reach a worldwide audience, in no small part due to the rapid and stratospheric rise of our YouTube channel (which you can find at YouTube.com/@HT-physio/).

But with great reach comes great responsibility. With each passing week, I couldn't help but feel that the initial publication of *Thriving Beyond Fifty* was not the best possible work I could produce. While the book largely received positive feedback, I felt some sections of it were lacking in detail and clarity on certain important issues. In hindsight, there were parts of the book I left light on information, and others in which I gave advice that I no longer follow in my own clinic.

A lot has changed since the first edition of this book went to print. There is new evidence on the optimal human diet for a start, which is a key area I look to address in this updated edition. My own understanding has changed greatly, too. I feel I am now able to synthesize my experience more succinctly into strategies that actually work for a huge number of conditions. I have tried to deliver more of these strategies in this new edition.

Some people mentioned how my pictures could have been clearer in the past editions of *Thriving Beyond Fifty*. This is something else that I have updated in the book you are holding, with every picture retaken to improve clarity.

I have tried to tackle almost all the conditions with which I am qualified to help people in this book. That is why the word count runs to 30 percent more than the previous edition, despite extensive editing for brevity. This has culminated in 25 additional chapters. I am proud of these new chapters and am certain they will help a great many people.

I once read that it takes 20 times the effort to write a 9-out-of-10 book as it does to write a 7-out-of-10 book. The effort required is non-linear, yet the impact the 9-out-of-10 book can have is disproportionately high. It is not my place to say whether or not this book has achieved that status. However, I can confidently say that the pages you are about to read are my very best effort to do so.

To encourage you to start your journey I've created a free downloadable guide: *The Top 5 Exercises for Over-50s Who Want to Remain Strong, Mobile & Active*. It is a roadmap to achieving strength, mobility and health and just requires a little effort on your part. Visit my site (**www.ht-physio.co.uk/guide**) to download this valuable guide for free. If you are serious about improving your strength, mobility and independence, you can also join my Lifelong Mobility™ program. Inside this special members' area you'll find my best exercise routines and other specially created content to help you improve your health that can't be found anywhere else. Find out more at **www.willharlow.com/lifelong**.

I hope you enjoy *Thriving Beyond Fifty*, and I ask of you one final favor if you do: share the book with someone else who you think might benefit from it. Thank you for trusting me with the investment of time it takes to read this book and I hope I can return your investment tenfold in the benefits it has on your health, now and in years to come.

Will Harlow

Introduction

First things first, I want to say well done for picking up this book. By reaching for it, then reading and applying the information within it, you'll be taking a significant step toward improving your health, both in body and mind.

As the author of *Thriving Beyond Fifty*, my promise to you is that, even if you only apply *one* suggestion or piece of advice from the following pages, you'll discover noticeable health benefits that will stand you in better stead for facing the next 10, 20 or 30 years ahead. Though this book is not designed to be the sole solution for any specific health problem or to provide you with any kind of diagnosis, the information within it can help you to stay healthy and happy, while avoiding the most common problems I see people suffering with every day.

If we don't know one another, I am the clinic owner and lead physiotherapist at my practice in Surrey, UK, called HT Physio. I set up the practice to help people over fifty years of age to overcome painful problems, avoid unnecessary surgeries and get back to living their active lives. You can read more about my practice and what I do by visiting https://ht-physio.co.uk.

I wrote this book for people who know there is still *so much living* to do after the fifty-year mark. I like to think of fifty as the halfway point in life; living to 100 years old may seem far-fetched, but getting there is becoming more and more realistic with each passing decade. The problem, though, is this: many people may live to a wonderful age in numerical terms, yet their later years are plagued by suffering and pain. This can turn the final decades of your life from being potentially the most rewarding to the most cruel and painful. I believe we should be exploring the world and enjoying each day after retirement; yet many of us end up slowing down, forced into a sedentary life through poor health.

In my eyes, living with daily pain is no way to exist and certainly shouldn't be seen as inevitable as we get older.

Of course, I'm not suggesting that it's possible to grow old without suffering any pain whatsoever; our biology is working against us in some respects. However, many of the problems I see every day and help people recover from are genuinely both preventable and treatable.

The sad truth is that many people I meet have suffered for far too long with a painful problem, simply because they accepted that this is the way it must be. If I achieve nothing else with this book than to encourage a belief in you that it is possible to improve the outlook of any long-standing painful problem you may be currently experiencing, then I will be content.

An additional aim with this book is to challenge the way we think about what our bodies can do as we get older. We automatically assume that a 25-year-old should be able to lift a suitcase or pick up a small child—but why do we accept the fact that only a handful of eighty-year-olds should be able to do the same? Of course, there's no denying the fact that muscles atrophy and lose strength as we age, and some of our joints will inevitably show signs of wear and tear, but these problems alone don't automatically determine whether or not we will be capable of performing physical tasks when we're older. In my opinion, we can strive to stay fit, healthy and strong as we get to eighty years old and beyond . . . but we *must* start now. This is backed by a growing body of research that swells year on year.

In the first section of this book, I discuss the fundamentals of strength, mobility and aging, and show you how to challenge the "inevitable" process of age-related deterioration that occurs in many . . . but not in all. My challenge for you is to strive to be in that smaller group, the group that defies the aging process, remaining fit and capable through their advancing years, despite the so-called odds being stacked against them.

How to Read This Book

If you're like me and you believe we should take care of our health as if it's our most valuable asset, then I know you'll enjoy the contents of this book and find the information useful. Because health is such a wide-ranging topic, I've written *Thriving Beyond Fifty* in a way that will be digestible for the reader who wishes to read it straight through, cover to cover. I have split it into several sections—separating the body into its respective parts—to help you navigate your way through the pages and pick the parts of the book that are most relevant to you, if you so wish. If you prefer to flick from section to section, I strongly recommend keeping a finger on the table of contents, using this as a reference point if you want to read the parts relevant to you. I would, however, suggest reading this book in its entirety if you have the time. You may find some nuggets of wisdom and information you can apply to your life right away, even in the chapters that you didn't expect to be applicable to you.

Within each chapter, I've attempted to unpick the reasons behind, as well as the solutions for, the most common health problems people face that are either preventable or treatable. You'll learn how to prevent and treat more than one type of shoulder pain. You'll read how arthritis may not necessarily be inevitable and how all hope is not lost if you've got the early signs already. You'll learn how not to fall (so you minimize the chance of lengthy hospital stays). I'll even show you some compelling evidence for techniques to mitigate the risk of dementia and depression, a feat once thought impossible.

I've attempted to back up all the information provided with scientific evidence wherever possible; you will find a reference list at the end of this book if you wish to peruse further or check my facts. I also wanted to include a free, yet incredibly valuable, resource for the readers of this book. You can learn more about that later or, if you simply cannot wait, turn to page 413 to find out more.

The first of my two requests of you, dear reader, is that you approach the information in these pages with an open mind. You may read some things that surprise you, or that challenge the beliefs you currently hold. That is OK; I'm not asking you to change your opinions or blindly believe my writing, just that you weigh up the evidence and the information I present, and then make up your own mind. My second request is that, if the information I present in this book sits well with you and you've got the "all clear" from your doctor, you apply it to your own life.

However, before applying any of the information in these pages, it is important that you seek advice from your doctor. As it is unlikely that we know each other, you must always get approval from your doctor before implementing anything you read in this book. There is a clearly labeled disclaimer in the following section which I advise you to read before continuing with the book.

Your health is your greatest asset. We only get one chance at living a long, healthy, comfortable life. My objective with this book is to give you some tools to improve yours.

Important Information

Throughout this book, you'll read about information, techniques and exercises (henceforth referred to as "strategies") I've used with my clients to help them improve certain aspects of their health or fitness. These strategies should not be taken as medical advice and should never be used as a substitute for individual medical advice from your doctor or the healthcare professionals involved in your care.

You shouldn't put into action any of the strategies from this book without first consulting your doctor about whether or not the strategies are suitable for your personal circumstances. Therefore, please check with your doctor before you put any of the strategies into action.

If you do choose to follow any of the strategies in this book, you do so at your own risk. While I have made every effort to ensure the strategies I recommend are safe, there will always be people who will not benefit from certain strategies given here. Therefore, use your own sense and judgement when deciding whether the strategies presented here are suitable for you. Not every strategy in this book will be suitable for every person.

Making changes to your health or exercise regime carries risks, including, but not limited to, worsening of your condition, sustaining injury or failing to achieve the results you set out to achieve. Please, therefore, weigh up all pros and cons with your own doctor before putting any strategies into action.

Please be aware that no strategy is 100 percent successful with everyone. I cannot guarantee your success if you choose to follow the strategies within this book. Please also be aware that there exists no provider–patient relationship established between the reader and the author as you work through this book, as this is only possible when the advice is tailored toward the patient, which this book is definitely not. Never disregard any advice from your doctor or healthcare professional because of something you read in this book. Do not use the information in this book as a substitute for diagnosis or treatment of any medical condition.

Part One

CRACKING
THE
FUNDAMENTALS

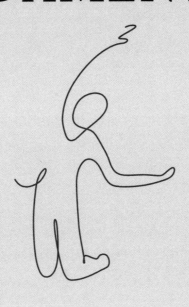

Common Terms

Before we dive into this book, I want to provide you with a short summary of the common terms I use in the text. I've tried not to let the "curse of knowledge" from my years of practice as a physiotherapist make my writing confusing. However, if you come across a term or phrase that you are unsure about, please rest assured that is my fault and not yours. Where possible, I have tried to explain terms and phrases as we go through the book, but this section may help you further. Think of it as a point of reference if you ever find yourself unclear.

Arthritis: Arthritis, or osteoarthritis, is a process characterized by the loss of cartilage in a joint, thickening of the underlying bone, the formation of tiny cysts in the bones and general deterioration of a moveable joint in the body. Despite common belief, pain from arthritis is NOT an inevitable part of aging. Many people have arthritis yet experience no pain whatsoever. It isn't clear why some people suffer so badly while others do not, but strength and mobility are crucial factors.

Bone: The strong structures that make up your skeleton, primarily made of collagen (a protein that provides a soft framework) and calcium (a mineral that hardens and strengthens the bone).

Cardiovascular training: A type of exercise with the goal of improving endurance as well as lung and heart health. Cardiovascular training doesn't make your muscles strong, but it does make your heart strong, with you becoming fitter as a result.

Cartilage: The cushioning and lubricating material that sits within every joint, between our bones. Cartilage allows normal, pain-free movement of our joints.

Cervical: In the context of this book, the term cervical means "to do with the neck." You have seven bones in your neck, called the cervical vertebrae.

Core: When we mention the term "core," we are referring to the muscle group in our abdomen that acts like a corset to keep our mid-section stable when we walk, sit and move. Without a core, you'd be a floppy disaster. We all have a core, but the core strength of two people might vary greatly (usually due to training, or a lack thereof).

Disc: The intervertebral discs sit between every vertebra in the spine. They comprise an outer sac that holds a jelly-like liquid in the interior. A disc prolapse (colloquially known as a "slipped disc") is a type of injury where the jelly-like substance pushes out of the disc and can irritate a nerve.

Endurance: The "staying power" you have in your heart, lungs and muscles during physical exercise. The better your endurance, the longer you can go on. Endurance is a comparable measure to the fuel economy in your car.

Exercise: Any activity you carry out with the express goal of getting fitter, stronger or more mobile.

Flexibility: Describes how flexible a muscle or joint is. Flexibility is subtly different to mobility in that it describes how much movement there is about a joint, regardless of control. I meet some patients who have tremendous flexibility (for example, they can bend forward and put their hands flat on the floor) but terrible control over that movement, rendering it unsafe. It is possible to have good flexibility but poor mobility.

General activity: The amount of movement you carry out in any given day as part of your normal, daily routine.

Inflammation: A natural process that occurs within the human body whereby certain chemicals are released by the blood vessels, causing swelling and pain. Inflammation isn't always bad; it is a natural response to injury and adaptation. However, it can be problematic when it runs amok (*more on this on pages 276–280*).

Joint: An area where a bone meets another bone. A joint is formed when ligaments attach two bones together and the two or more bones articulate with one another. In a healthy situation, the bones that make up a joint are lined with cartilage, which is a cushion that prevents bones from rubbing together. Joints allow movement; muscles either side of the joint pull on a bone to produce motion. We have a variety of different joints in our body, including hinge joints (such as the knee) and ball-and-socket joints (such as the shoulder).

Ligament: A ligament is a fibrous band that joins bone to bone. Ligaments are strong bands of collagen and are much simpler in their composition compared to a tendon. You can think of ligaments as the parcel tape that keeps a box in shape. We have ligaments securing every joint in our body.

Lumbar: This refers to your lower back. In your lumbar region, you have five vertebrae. They are the biggest vertebrae in the spine. There should be a natural curve in the lumbar spine called a lordosis, which is the opposite of a kyphosis. If this curve becomes too great, it can cause problems.

Mobility: Discussed in two contexts. First, mobility can refer to how well you can generally get about on your feet, or up and down from a chair. This can be called "general mobility." Second, mobility can refer to the movement capacity and control of a specific joint. This can be called "movement-specific mobility." Think of the term "mobility" in both senses to describe how well one can move.

Mobility training: A type of exercise with the goal of improving the capacity for movement and control around a joint or area of the body. This could include certain types of stretching, but gaining control of these new ranges of motion is the most important part of mobility exercises.

Muscle: The fleshy parts of our body that contract to produce movement. Muscles contract and, when they do, they pull on a bony attachment. This pulls one bone toward another, thus producing movement. One important fact: muscles cannot push, only pull.

Muscle imbalance: We always have more than one muscle at work around any given joint in the body. Usually, muscles work as a team; one muscle might stabilize the joint, while the other contracts to produce movement. However, this process can sometimes go wrong and cause a problem with motion, often leading to pain. This is referred to as a "muscle imbalance." They can often go unnoticed for many years before seeming "suddenly" to lead to a painful problem. Muscle imbalances can cause pain through an accumulation of stress on the joints, even without any obvious injury.

Nerve: The two-way channels that carry messages from our brain to our limbs and muscles (or vice versa), telling them to move after the brain initiates the message. Nerves also transmit the signals that cause us to experience pain.

Power: A function of strength and speed. Power is calculated by multiplying the strength of a muscle contraction by how quickly that contraction can be produced. An example of a powerful movement would be a jump, requiring a rapid and considerable contraction of the leg muscles.

Resistance training: A type of exercise with the goal of strengthening a group of muscles in the body. This could include weightlifting or body-weight exercises like push-ups.

Spine: The bony part of your back and neck. We have 24 moveable bones in the spine (called vertebrae), plus a sacrum and a coccyx (the two bones that make up your bottom and "tail" area).

Strength: The ability to generate force using the muscles. In general, having greater strength is almost always a positive thing. This is why I speak about the importance of getting strong many times in this book. You can find a free gift to help you with this goal on page 413.

Tendon: A rope-like structure that joins a muscle to a bone. While these structures may look like a simple piece of rope to the untrained eye, they are very complex, composed of many different types of cells (their complexity is one reason why they can become problematic).

Thoracic: This term refers to your mid back. You have 12 thoracic vertebrae. There should be a natural curve in the thoracic spine, called a kyphosis. If the curve becomes too extreme, it can cause problems, like a hunched back.

The Process of Aging

All plants and animals age with each passing year. Humans are no different. While we all have a good idea what aging looks like for many people, why do these physical changes occur? And why do some people look and feel far older than others, despite being the same age?

The visible and internal effects of aging occur due to the process that the cells in our body undergo with each passing year. The cells in our body multiply to replace old cells at different rates; some replicate very frequently (such as skin cells) while others are hardly replaced at all (such as brain cells). Each cell has a finite number of times that it can replicate to produce a brand new cell. Once it reaches this limit, the cell dies and is reabsorbed by the body. As these cells are lost or damaged, the process of aging starts to show.

Our skin starts to become thinner and show wrinkles as a result of a steady loss of skin cells. The surface of our skin becomes visibly drier as we produce less sweat and oil as we age. Under the skin, our bones become more pronounced as we store less fat in these visible areas. The rate of bone loss accelerates to outweigh the rate of bone growth occurring in our bodies. Our muscles lose mass and strength, meaning we can't run, jump or lift as easily as we once could.

But it's not all doom and gloom! With age comes wisdom, different perspectives and a wealth of experience. What's more, some aging processes can be mitigated—and some can be reversed. With effort and the right regime, it is possible for older individuals to reverse the rate of muscle loss within their body and actually become stronger. I have seen it with my own eyes on many occasions. The first and biggest step is accepting that it is possible and that a slow, aging decline is not inevitable.

One of the reasons aging happens seemingly so quickly for many people is that they succumb to the temptation to make life easier by design as they grow older. Gradually decreasing their activity levels with each passing year, as family members constantly remind them to "take it easy," they lose vital steps each day. If you choose to become more sedentary over time, you'll gradually lose the ability to carry out the key fundamental human movements without even realizing it. Once you lose the ability to perform these fundamental movements, there will likely be situations where you'll need the assistance of others. You'll live with a higher risk of injury and your mobility and independence could even be threatened in advancing years.

I don't wish this loss of mobility and independence on anyone. This is why I've laid out the movements I believe to be key for over-fifties (the "Nine at Ninety") to protect and maintain vitality as the years advance. With some awareness, persistence and discipline, it's possible to practice and regain these movements should you find that you struggle to perform them as well as you'd like. You can find these fundamental movements on pages 20–33.

The other part of us that can be affected by aging is the brain. It is a common misconception that problems such as dementia and Alzheimer's disease (AD) are directly caused by the aging process. Dementia and AD are *not normal* human processes and we shouldn't just expect and accept that they are a fact of life. In this book, we'll talk about strategies for keeping the brain, and the mind it contains, young and nimble.

Research carried out over the last 50 years has unearthed the fact that our fate is not entirely dictated by a predetermined destiny. Major causes of death and disability, such as AD, once considered part of the genetic lottery, have been exposed as, to some extent, a result of the way we live our lives. This growing body of research is monumentally exciting; it puts our destinies back into our hands. For example, one of the key mitigating factors against AD isn't a pill or medication, but exercise. We will talk about the positive effects of exercise, which are simply too compelling to ignore.

So, while aging was once regarded as simply the inevitable process of moving closer and closer to the grave, we can now view it in a different, modern, more informed and hopeful way. It is important to realize that we have a choice as to how we live through the aging process. We truly can control aging when it comes to our health, fitness and mobility, and the aging process of our brains is largely within our control too. This mindset may be one of the most important shifts you'll need to make to get the most out of this book.

Once you have internalized the fact that you do have a choice when it comes to how growing old feels, looks and plays out for you, you'll feel empowered to start making positive changes. And maybe you'll stop rolling your eyes and saying, "I guess I'm just getting old," whenever you get a new ache or pain!

What Is Mobility?

Mobility is the term given to two different aspects of your physical health. One definition of mobility is simply how well you can move about. Having good mobility means you can get out of a low chair, climb stairs, and even adjust your feet quickly to react to a trip more easily than someone with poor mobility.

The second definition of mobility is body-area specific. This type of mobility refers to how well you can control the movement of a particular joint throughout its complete range of motion. For example, you may be able to raise your arms over your head, but how stable are you when you get there? Do you have enough control to perform an intricate task, like changing a light bulb? Having control throughout a range of motion is one of the most important parts of injury prevention and something we will talk about a lot throughout the course of this book.

Both types of mobility are crucial to leading a long, happy, healthy life. Of course, they both feed into one another. Maintaining the ability to get about is only possible when you have good control through the joints in your lower limbs. Maintaining this good range of motion is only possible when you remain active and regularly use the movement capabilities available to you. We're going to call the first type of mobility "general mobility"—the ability to get about easily. The second type of mobility is "movement-specific mobility"—the ability to control the movement of a specific part of your body.

How do you know whether you have good general mobility?

The answer to this question really lies in what you'd like to be able to do in terms of movement each day. Good mobility for someone who works an active job and likes to take long walks at the weekend might look different to good mobility for an 86-year-old who just wants to be able to collect their paper from the shop every morning.

If you want to assess or improve your mobility, the first thing you should do is to write down what you'd like to be able to achieve each day without pain, feeling tired or feeling the need to stop when you're out and about. For example, you might decide that you want to be able to take the dog out for a 20-minute walk each morning, get into the gym three times each week, and be able to go for a two-hour walk every weekend without having to crash on Sunday because you're so worn out. Start by writing down the activities you'd like to be able to achieve each week. Be specific with distance and duration.

Once you have your list, I want you to write down what you're currently doing each week in terms of general activity. Look at the two lists and compare. You may currently be doing 70 percent of what you'd like to be able to do. This is fine; simply make a resolution for yourself, starting right now, that each week you're going to add 5 percent to your total activity level, until you reach your general mobility goal.

You may already be at 100 percent of your general mobility goal. This is also fine; make a resolution to continue with this level of general mobility, and when you feel it slipping, you'll know to take action early, as opposed to being oblivious to your mobility levels as they slip away. As you'll now be more aware of your activity levels, you'll be able to tot up a total of your weekly activity and compare it to your goals. If you miss a dog walk one morning, you'll know you're only at 95 percent for your general mobility quota that week, so you might add another 20 minutes onto your long walk on the weekend. There are endless ways to make up the general mobility quota you set for yourself; it just takes a little planning and preparation to do so.

How do you know whether you have good movement-specific mobility?

It's possible to assess the movement-specific mobility of every single joint in the body, and this is something I do regularly with my clients in my clinic. However, for the purpose of this section of the book, we will focus on testing your shoulder, hip, knee and ankle mobility. If you feel that you lack mobility in these or in other areas of the body, you will be able to find some guidance on how to improve these sticky areas elsewhere in this book.

- For the shoulder, you should be able to lift your arms high above your head without pain and without arching your back. You should also be able to reach up behind your back as far as your shoulder blade, as if to reach for a bra strap. Going in the other direction, you should be able to touch the back of your head with ease while letting your elbow roll out. If any of these movements are tricky for you, you may lack shoulder mobility.

- For the hip, you should have no trouble putting your shoes and socks on. Getting in and out of a car should be easy without having to turn your body and "reverse" back into the seat. If you have difficulty getting in and out of cars (especially low ones), or need to use a shoehorn to put on your shoes, your hip mobility may be poor. A bit of effort to improve it would help to safeguard this area of your body from future problems.

- For your knees, you should be able to squat down and pick something up from the floor by bending your knees, without having to rely on bending at the waist. When sat on a sofa with your legs up on the seat stretched out in front of you, you should be able to lock your knees out so that they are fully straight. If there's a slight bend in the knee when you do try to lock the knee out, you may lack full extension of the knee joint. This can lead to problems with walking.

- Finally, for your ankles, you should be able to squat so your thighs are parallel to the floor without your heels lifting up from the ground. If you can't do this because your ankles or calves are stiff and tight, it can change the entire mechanics of this very common movement and put undue stress through various parts of the body, including the knees and spine.

It's worth taking the time to test the mobility of each of these joints in turn, being careful as you do so. If you find any pain, stiffness or tightness, don't worry—none of us is perfect—but you should certainly make a commitment to put in the work to improve the movement-specific mobility of this area of your body. Your body is one of your greatest assets and you need to make sure you look after it; after all, you only get one!

What Is Strength?

Throughout this book, one of the attributes we're going to talk about, possibly more than any other, is strength. By strength, I'm referring to the capability of a group of muscles within your body to produce force and therefore movement. Without strength, movement is impossible.

Strength is key, especially for the over-fifties. Being strong protects you from injury, as your joints will be far better supported against the effects of gravity. You'll be less likely to experience pain with arthritis. You'll be far less likely to fall or to suffer a life-changing injury as a result. You'll feel safer when you're out of the house and your confidence will grow as a result. You'll be able to do more around the home without worrying about paying for it the next day.

There really are no downsides to being strong, and one of the greatest gifts I can give to my clients is when I help them get strong enough to cope with the demands of their active lives.

So, how much strength do you really need to be healthy, fit and to remain active past the age of fifty? There are individual factors, including your daily routine, hobbies and goals, which determine the answer to this question. However, everyone needs a base level of strength to cope with the daily demands of life, unless you plan on becoming a couch potato until you pass away!

Being able to lift a small suitcase over your head is a great indicator of upper-body strength for over-fifties. If you can carry out this task without undue stress or strain—necessary when you board the plane bound for your next holiday, of course—it's likely that you've got good strength in your arms and shoulders.

Being able to go from standing to sitting in a low chair very slowly, without using your hands or letting yourself "drop" the last 7cm (3in) into the chair, is a fantastic indicator of lower-body strength. Although most of us get up and down from chairs every single day, it's incredible how much we use our upper body without realizing in order to help us, sparing our legs . . . *and* causing them to become weaker as a result. We are also inclined to drop quickly into chairs, relinquishing control to gravity, which causes us to quickly lose control.

You should also have no problem walking on your tiptoes if asked to do so. This action proves lower-body strength and demonstrates strong and capable feet and ankles.

These movements are some of the key indicators I use to test the strength of my clients. If they struggle to carry out these common, everyday actions when aged fifty-five, how hard is life going to be at eighty?

But if you can't complete these actions without stress and strain on your body, it's not too late to do something about it. While muscle mass may continue to be lost with each advancing year, strength can be gained and maintained through practice and commitment. My aim is to show you how to do exactly that in this book. You can also find some fantastic additional resources to help you build strength in the Resources section on page 413 of this book.

What Is Endurance?

Endurance is your staying power. Having substantial endurance is a prerequisite for being able to participate in daily life. If you have poor endurance, it's impossible to walk, run or cycle as far as you'd like. Endurance is determined by how efficient your lungs and heart are, as well as how much capacity for repetitive work exists within your muscles.

But why is endurance important?

Well, for a start, it determines how far you're able to walk with friends and family. It dictates how much of the housework you can get done in any given period. It also determines how likely you are to suffer an injury (to a certain extent) and can even be used to predict the cardiovascular health of an individual and the consequential likelihood of a heart attack.

While endurance usually refers to cardiovascular activity (the type of exercise that gets the heart pumping and the lungs working hard), we can also apply it to daily tasks, such as building a new piece of furniture or even cleaning your house.

A key point to consider about endurance is that it is very task-specific. For example, if you were to take a marathon runner, who is incredibly fit and has excellent running endurance, and put them on a bike, you might be surprised at how poorly they perform. The same is true for us and our daily tasks. We become very efficient at the things we do often—but not quite so good at new tasks that we don't know well, even if those tasks look simple at first glance.

How much endurance is enough to live a healthy life? The answer to this question is determined by your daily routine and the way you choose to live your life. Someone who runs three times per week will need more endurance than someone who just wants to maintain their garden. However, it is important to ensure that you maintain a baseline level of fitness that is sufficient for you to cope with the stresses and strains of daily life.

One way to improve your endurance is simply to add a little more activity onto the end of what you normally do, each time you do it. Endurance is built progressively and very slowly, just like building strength by working a specific muscle over and over again. If you want to be fitter so you can walk further or get more done each day, you need first to work out how much you can already do within your current capacity. How much activity does it take until you feel like you have to stop, or until you're out of breath? This is your current endurance capacity.

If you want to improve your endurance capacity, the most sensible protocol goes something like this: next time you're out walking or doing jobs around the home, add five minutes onto the end of what you'd normally do before stopping. When you feel the call of a sit-down on the sofa and a cup of tea, spur yourself on to do just five more minutes. If you're walking, take a slightly longer route than you normally would, but one that adds no more than five minutes onto your total walking time. Alternatively, you could try to walk roughly 5 percent more quickly than the speed at which you usually do.

By adding five extra minutes or 5 percent more effort to your current level of activity, you can slowly and incrementally build your staying power so that it's there to call on in the future, when you may absolutely need it. Having a solid level of endurance might be the difference between catching that flight and missing it altogether if you happen to be caught in awful traffic on the way to the airport. It might be the difference between getting across the road safely and stumbling as you reach the other side. It might be the difference between a happy, tail-wagging pup and a sulking so-and-so after you tell the poor dog you can't take him out for a walk tonight because you're *just too tired*.

Building endurance takes time and a concerted effort, but once you start to reap the rewards, you'll feel such a difference. Imagine being able to climb that hill without getting out of breath; getting to the top of a long flight of stairs without feeling like your heart is going to burst out of your chest; or getting to the end of the day and feeling tired—but far from exhausted. These are the pay-offs for your hard work.

You'll also find benefits that aren't necessarily detectable by you, but which will make a huge difference to your health. An improvement in heart health can lead to a dramatic decrease in the likelihood of suffering a fatal heart attack. It can prevent build-up of plaque in your arteries that could lead to a catastrophic event like a stroke. Improving your endurance is like taking out an insurance policy on your overall health. Being fitter is directly correlated with a reduced risk not just of cardiovascular problems, but of certain types of cancer and even brain disorders such as dementia.[1, 2]

So, the next time you're out for that weekend walk, try pushing yourself a little bit harder. Your heart, lungs and indeed the rest of your entire body will thank you for it.

Key Fundamental Movements (the Nine at Ninety!)

When you consider the things we have to do every day, there are a handful of common, yet highly challenging, movements we need to perform on a regular basis. After careful deliberation, I've compiled a list of the nine movements that I feel everyone should still be able to perform at age ninety.

If you have the ability to do every one of these activities without pain or restriction, it'll be unlikely that you'll be faced with anything in day-to-day life that you cannot handle. So, in no particular order, here are the nine key fundamental human movements—the Nine at Ninety—which, if maintained throughout your life, will give you the best chance of a healthy body and incredible longevity, and make no physical challenge insurmountable.

1. The Chair Squat (with Load)

This is an action we perform every single day, multiple times, yet most of us find incredibly imaginative ways to cheat. This causes us to miss out on the benefits of performing the action properly, and we lose the ability to perform it easily when required, as a result. What movement am I talking about? Getting in and out of a chair, of course!

Common cheating patterns usually appear in two ways:

- Using our hands as leverage on well-placed chair arms

- Dropping into the chair on the way down

So, as the first fundamental movement, my challenge to you is to be able to sit down and stand up from a low chair, one that puts your knees at a 90-degree angle when sitting, without the use of your hands. To make things harder but more effective, you're going to do so while holding something in front of your body. The reason you'll be holding something (preferably with a load of around 10 percent of your body weight) in front of your body is to add resistance—as well as to busy your hands and prevent you from reaching for those chair arms!

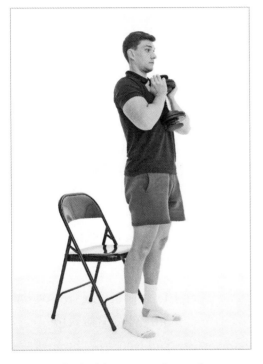

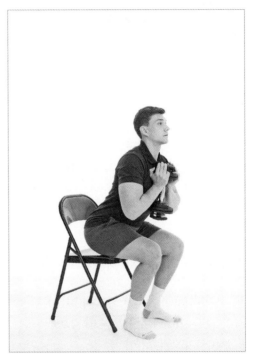

1. Begin by holding a small weight in front of your body, close to your chest. Stand with the backs of your legs in contact with the seat of the chair.

2. Bending at the hips and the knees but keeping a straight spine, slowly (to the count of four seconds) lower yourself onto the chair. Be sure to avoid 'dropping' onto the chair at the final moment!

Why This Movement Is Key

Being able to sit down and stand up with good control throughout this motion, without using your hands, shows excellent control of your thigh muscles—one of the key muscle groups for many tasks we perform every day. I use this movement as my number one quick screening tool when I have a client with a lower-limb problem, to check how well they're moving before we get to work.

2. The Suitcase Lift

Going on vacation can be wonderful and something we look forward to for many months prior to the trip. But traveling can bring about a host of challenges that we don't often face at other times of the year. One such challenge is lugging about a heavy suitcase, especially if you're going away for a period longer than one week.

We are forced to maneuver our suitcases in various ways around the airport and into transfer vehicles, which can be made easier by readily available assistance. However, one task that many of my clients hate relinquishing to others is the job of depositing the carry-on luggage into the overhead storage compartment on an airplane. Passing the task of lifting your wife's suitcase to the young buck in the seat behind, in front of a plane full of people, can feel embarrassing.

By building enough strength to ensure you can complete this action, you're not only able to maintain your own independence in these matters but also help others less fortunate with their physical capabilities than you are. Suddenly, you'll transform into the one eagerly offering help to the cabin around you and not paying for it the next day.

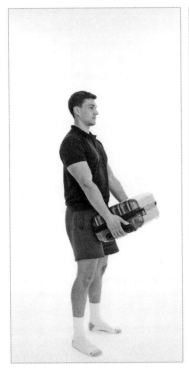 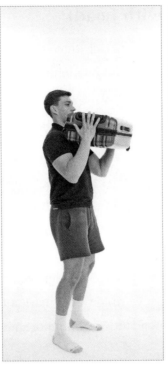 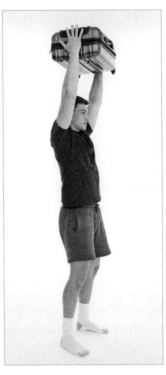

1. Lift a suitcase from the floor, using your legs as opposed to your back. Rest the suitcase against the front of your legs.

2. Use the strength in your arms and shoulders to bring the suitcase to chest height.

3. Keeping your buttocks squeezed tightly to protect your back, extend your arms and lift the suitcase overhead.

Why This Movement Is Key

Being able to lift your luggage over your head and deposit it safely and securely, then retrieve it upon landing, is a feat that requires considerable upper-body strength and stability. The shoulders, arms and "core" muscles are all highly active when we lift and shift above our heads, and excellent shoulder mobility is also required when it comes to reaching for your case. If you can lift a heavy case overhead in a tightly packed airplane and stow it away safely, there probably aren't many overhead tasks in daily life that will cause you a great deal of trouble.

3. The Stair Climb (with Load)

For most people, stairs are a daily obstacle that we are forced to navigate. This is a good thing: stairs keep our legs strong and our joints mobile. I always fear for my clients when they downgrade from a house to a bungalow, as they'll lose the 10-plus trips up the stairs each day and miss out on clocking up valuable minutes of strengthening exercise as a result.

However, being able to climb the stairs is only half the battle. It's important to be able to climb the stairs without the use of the handrail when one isn't available. It's also important to be able to transport a heavy load in each hand up and down the staircase when required. A great example of a load that we have to transfer regularly up and down stairs are bags of heavy shopping. We might buy a new lamp or want to decorate the bedroom, for example, or we might even have an upstairs kitchen. Either way, carrying a load upstairs independently is an important job we regularly have to do.

Why This Movement Is Key

If you think about the way we climb stairs, we must put all of our weight on one leg when we transfer from one step to another. This requires balance and single-leg stability, which is vital for many of our other daily tasks. We also need to use our thigh muscles to their maximum capability to control our descent down a flight of stairs, more so than when we walk on the flat. Climbing the stairs with a bag of shopping in each hand is a great acid test for your leg strength and overall stability. If you can do this task, it should bring you confidence across the board.

4. The Floor Get-Up

One of the things I am most proud of when it comes to the treatment I offer in my clinic is that I regularly help my clients to avoid the terrifying prospect of a fall. Falling can be catastrophic for anyone, but especially for people over the age of seventy. In the

UK, falls cost the National Health Service over £2 billion per year, purely due to the extent of the physical damage that can occur from the impact. Coupled with the fact that fallers are more likely to have fragile bones than the general population, the perils of suffering a fall are enormous and should be prevented at all costs where possible.

However, most of us will fall at some stage in our lives. Luckily, for many people falls don't damage anything more than their confidence, but having fallen there is another problem you must face. That problem is how to get up from the floor, especially when no one else is around.

The NHS guidelines, taught to us in my hospital placement days, recommended the use of a chair to pull on to go from lying to kneeling, then the use of that same chair to push up onto to go from kneeling to standing. However, what happens when there are no chairs or other suitable pieces of furniture within reach? I've met more than one older person who has fallen in their home, and despite not being injured, has had to wait for paramedics to arrive before they have been able to get back onto their feet. This has been a particularly distressing event for each of these people, and I wouldn't wish it on anyone.

That is why I believe being able to get up from the floor, without the use of a chair or any other piece of furniture to help, is one of the essential and fundamental movements that make up my Nine at Ninety. It is also the movement that may be considered the hardest of the nine movements, involving literally the entire body and a series of complex and coordinated actions.

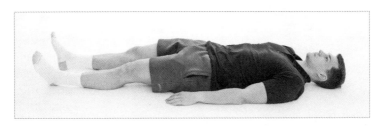

1. Begin by lying flat on the floor.

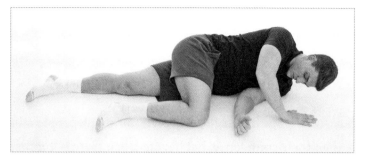

2. Bend your right knee so that your right foot is flat on the floor, then swing your right leg over your left leg, using the momentum to turn onto your left side.

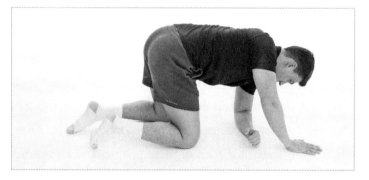

3. Using your arms for stability, continue turning your body, bending your left knee as you do so, until you are in a kneeling position.

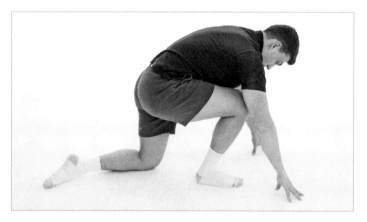

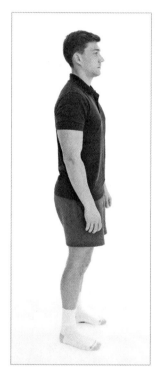

5. Move your right leg forward and place your right foot on the floor, then push back with your hands to slowly straighten into a standing position.

4. Continue to bring the leg through and place the foot on the floor, then rise to a kneeling position.

Why This Movement Is Key

We've discussed why being able to get up from the floor is so critical, but what does it actually take to be able to get up and down from the floor? For a start, you need impressive "core" strength: the capability of your midriff to stabilize your body as you move through the steps from lying to kneeling and then standing. Once in a kneeling position, it takes a fair amount of leg strength to push up to standing without toppling over.

All in all, this is the ultimate movement—once you can achieve the floor get-up, you'll have impressive confidence and should find the other fundamental movements on this list a piece of cake in comparison.

One last word about practising this movement: I would suggest you start on a soft carpeted floor with someone supervising and plenty of furniture within reach for use in helping you to stand up if you get stuck.

5. The Hole Dig

Is there any task in the garden more physical than digging a great big hole? Digging holes can be an incredibly satisfying activity and one that I always used to love on the rare occasions that I would help my mum in the garden.

Digging a hole isn't just a necessary part of transforming a garden, though; it's also a great marker of strength and endurance. Digging with a heavy spade is an activity that involves a range of muscle groups, meaning the benefits of this activity are widespread, too. You'll probably notice yourself getting breathless as you dig the hole. This shows how the cardiovascular system is also being called upon to join in and is strengthened as a result.

Why This Movement Is Key

When digging a hole, you'll need both upper- and lower-body strength. Not only will each thrust of the spade require a maximal effort from your muscles, but the effort will require your heart and lungs to be working well, too. Because of this, being able to dig a hole represents the ability to perform a truly practical, physical activity that transfers across many other DIY or garden tasks.

6. The Five-Mile Walk

So far, we've discussed movements that require a lot of explosive strength and impressive mobility. But what is the activity we do the most each day, which also happens to be the number one hobby of thousands of over-fifties? The answer to that question is: walking.

Being able to walk without discomfort is an absolute necessity for a happy, healthy life. Experts have long believed that getting 10,000 steps in each day (the truth about which comes later in the book) is an effective way of mitigating the risk of many health problems; but how many of us have the capacity to do that number of steps all in one go?

The ability to walk five miles is a great indicator of excellent general mobility and endurance. Being able to walk this far opens up a whole new list of possibilities for social activities, as well as giving you licence to explore some of the beautiful natural treats the countryside has to offer.

Why This Movement Is Key

You can think of walking over a medium-to-long distance as a good audit of your general mobility. Over this type of distance, little niggles and problems with your walking technique are likely to show—highlighting areas of your body that need extra work. What's more, having the ability to walk five miles gives you confidence in certain situations that, luckily, we don't have to contend with very often but are always a possibility, such as being stranded somewhere far-flung after your car has broken down, with no signal to call the breakdown services.

7. The Gardening Crouch

This movement isn't limited solely to the garden, although that is possibly the time when you'll need it most. The gardening crouch describes the process of squatting down and sitting back on your haunches in order to reach something low to the ground. You would also need this movement in situations such as reaching for something in a low cupboard in your kitchen. Imagine you have to pull up a weed from the ground, but you don't want to get your knees muddy. You're going to need to crouch down while remaining supported on two feet. This is the gardening crouch:

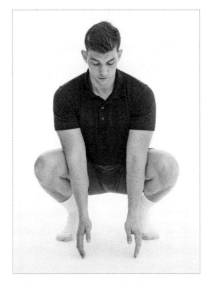
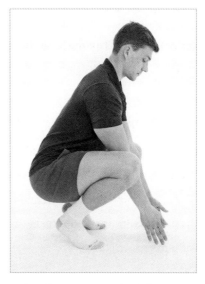

Gardening crouch, front view   Gardening crouch, side view

The gardening crouch is primarily a marker of good mobility. It requires excellent mobility of your ankles, knees and hips to be able to hold it comfortably. The common substitute people make for this movement when they lack proper mobility in their lower limbs is to "fold" at the waist and use the movement of their lower back to reach for the floor. While not necessarily harmful to do once or twice, constant repetitive use of this action can lead to back pain and isn't good for long-term back health.

Using the gardening crouch, your weight is going through your ankles, knees and hips, which are much better designed to tolerate the load of your body. The easiest way to tell whether or not you are capable of the gardening crouch is to think back to the last time you were transferring a small plant from a pot to the garden, or when you needed something out of a low cupboard—what did you do to get down there? Did you bend at the waist while keeping your legs straight? Did you sit on the floor? Did you go down onto your knees?

If you did any of those things instead of the gardening crouch, you may lack mobility in one or two of the key joints in your legs. Don't worry—we'll talk later in this book about how to improve the movement in those joints if they are indeed limited.

The Gardening Crouch involves near-maximal knee mobility, which may take time to regain.

Why This Movement Is Key

This movement is part of the Nine at Ninety because it demonstrates excellent hip, knee and ankle health. A person cannot put their entire body weight through their fully bent knees if their knees are deteriorated, stiff or unhealthy. While some strength is involved, this movement really tests the mobility of the lower limb, more so than the other movements on this list.

8. The Box Lift

Being able to pick up a heavy object from very low down on the floor is a vital ability to retain in advancing years. First, let's picture the movement: imagine a heavy box in your front room that needs moving into the kitchen. To pick it up you must bend down, at the waist and the knees, gripping the box around the lower edges, and then extend your back and knees so as to lift it up and carry it away.

To do so, you'll need sufficient grip strength to get started. Being able to use your fingers and hands effectively is incredibly important at any stage of your life. There are chapters on how to maintain the use of your hands later in this book.

You'll also need to use the proper lifting technique to perform this exercise well. There is, in fact, a "right" way to lift, a way that will use the full potential of your leg and back muscles while also mitigating the risk of injury. It's very important to use the strength in your back and legs to perform this movement properly, protecting your back while safely lifting the box into your arms.

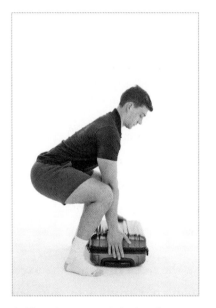 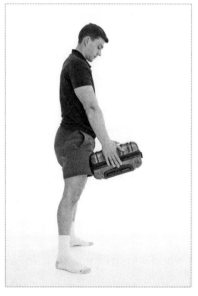

1. Keeping a straight back, bend at the hips and knees to bring your hands low enough so that they can get underneath the object.

2. Pushing up through the feet, extend the hips and knees while maintaining a straight back, and stand up with the object in your arms.

Why This Movement Is Key

We have to lift things from the floor quite often. Fortunately for us, most things that we lift are light and can be moved relatively safely, regardless of technique. However, when we come across a heavy load firmly planted on the floor that needs shifting, it's important we have the ability to do this without putting ourselves at risk of injury. For this movement, ankle and hip mobility are vital, as well as strength and coordination of the lower-limb muscles. Without all of these prerequisites, we'll be putting ourselves at unnecessary risk.

9. The Wood Chop

The final movement in the Nine at Ninety is one that not many of us have to do with any regularity, but one that highlights strength, stability and mobility almost better than any other.

This movement is the "wood chop." Think of a lumberjack chopping wood on a block, swinging an axe overhead and bringing it down with incredible accuracy onto a semi-split log. While I'm not suggesting that you go to a hardware store and purchase the largest axe you can find, some of you reading this chapter may still chop wood in this way. Even if you don't, I think it's important to consider just how many different areas of the body need to work in tandem to produce such a primal movement. Once you have a mental picture of the demands this task involves, you can decide whether it is something that is within your capability or not.

Chopping wood requires you first to generate the force to swing the axe with your lower limbs, then transfer the force up through your trunk into your arms, before contracting your shoulders and trunk to bring the axe down. In this way, almost every muscle group in the body is used in a chain reaction.

Why This Movement Is Key

As previously mentioned, this task isn't something most of us have to do very often, but it is a fantastic "movement audit" for the whole body. You'll need strength in both upper and lower limbs, as well as excellent mobility in the spine, hips and shoulders to perform this movement effectively. If you can safely chop wood at ninety and beyond, you'll be doing incredibly well!

What to Do With the Nine at Ninety

If you've considered the movements I describe above and think that most of these are within your capabilities at this current time, that's fantastic and should be applauded. Your task is simply to maintain your ability to perform these movements as each year passes, watching out for early signs of stiffness or weakness that may prohibit your movement.

Key "sticky" areas to watch for are loss of movement in your shoulder joints, tightness in your calves and stiffness in the hips and knees. Keep an eye on these areas and seek guidance if you feel stiffness or tightness setting in any time soon.

If you can't complete the tasks in the Nine at Ninety, don't worry: it's likely that you're just out of practice. When we don't use these parts of our body regularly, we lose the ability to call on them when we need to. But, in many cases, this process is reversible! With some targeted work or treatment from a skilled professional, there are many goals that are closer to being within reach than you think.

First, you need to work out if the reason that you can't perform these movements is because of lack of practice, or because of an injury preventing you from doing so. My recommendation would be to get the injury problem solved first before trying to push on with these tasks. Seek out some professional advice about your individual circumstances.

Once your injury has improved, look for the strength and mobility advice within this book, which will demonstrate the ways that you can improve your movement, taking you ever closer to being able to safely perform the Nine at Ninety.

One of the key things to remember is that improving strength and mobility takes a long time! You're likely to be several months, at a minimum, away from your goals. However, just a short period of time dedicated to solving these problems each day will go a long way to improving your capability in these actions and many more that you carry out each day.

The "Magic Formula" for Fixing Injuries

Throughout my time at university, I found the vague instructions for how to help someone recover from injury to be incredibly frustrating. I used to complain about the fact that we were never given clear, step-by-step instructions for rehabilitating a person. I craved a "formula," some kind of mental model I could hold in my mind and apply to my future patients.

I now understand that the lecturers were trying to encourage independent thinking, which is why such a formula was never taught. But now I have a decade of practice under my belt, I believe I have come close to discovering the closest thing to a formula that can help to relieve almost any injury. The formula is as follows:

- First, we must reduce pain. This might mean someone needs a few days of rest immediately following an injury, or a period of icing the area to bring down inflammation. This is also the time when hands-on treatment is often most effective, releasing tightness and easing pain.

- Once the pain has been reduced, the second step is to improve mobility. In the case of most injuries, range of motion around an affected joint will be adversely affected. This makes the area stiff and restricted. Gently encouraging the return of this range of motion is a vital next step. This can be done through gentle exercises, or through the help of manual treatment.

- The third step in the formula is to improve strength. After an injury, there is an inevitable loss of strength in the muscles around the affected region. It takes only two weeks for noticeable losses in muscle strength, meaning weakness sets in very quickly. The only way to regain strength is through strengthening exercises designed to activate the target muscles, improving both the function of the muscle fibers and the connection between the mind and the muscle.

- The fourth and final step is to restore full function. This is person- and injury-specific. If you are a golfer with a back injury, for example, this stage would mean gradually reintroducing the movements of a normal golf swing into your daily routine, in order to "reacclimatize" the body to performing these movements safely. If you are a walker with an Achilles tendon problem, this stage would mean gradually increasing your walking now the pain has reduced significantly. This stage also includes restoring balance, if this has been affected by the injury.

Where most people go wrong is they might jump from stage one straight to stage four. They rest their injury for a few days, then once the pain is gone they try to get back out on the golf course. The problem is, they are still lacking mobility and strength, so the injury inevitably returns. Show me someone who keeps suffering repeated injuries, and I'll show you someone who has never fully satisfied all four steps of the injury recovery process.

Throughout the rest of this book, I will show you in more detail how to follow the four stages of this process for many different injuries.

My Principles for Treating Physical Health Problems

People often ask me whether I have suffered any significant injuries in the past, and if so, how did I deal with them?

To tell you the truth, I had my fair share of injuries in my younger years, all of them related in some way or another to sports. Being keen on football, squash and weightlifting throughout my adolescence, I exposed my body to extremes of load, impact and volume. Inevitably, the constant stress and strain led me to suffer several injuries, with the worst being to my right shoulder.

During a game of football, my shoulder rolled out of the socket and then instantly back in, an injury we call a subluxation. This is like a minor version of a dislocation, yet it can cause just as many long-term problems. The issue following a subluxation is that the surrounding ligaments are permanently stretched, meaning the affected joint loses some of its fundamental stability. It took me a total of three years of rehabilitation to get my shoulder back to a point where I considered it "normal" again. Looking back, the principles I used to deal with my shoulder are the same I use today to help guide others' decisions about how to treat their own injuries and wider health problems.

My first principle when it comes to treating an illness or injury is to try to fix it through exercise. That might mean stretching, strengthening or mobilizing the affected area. With my shoulder, I put together a rehab program involving all of the above, dedicating about 15 to 30 minutes of focused exercise to the area every day.

Exercise can also help other problems, too. There is a large body of evidence to show that exercise can help to relieve not just physical but mental health issues as well. Therefore, the principle of starting with exercise applies to many different health problems about which I advise people.

However, exercise alone won't fix everything. In an ideal world, we could fix every problem with just exercise, without changing any other facet of our lives. Yet this is rarely possible. For that reason, if exercise alone doesn't work for fixing the problem at hand, I move on to the second principle, which is lifestyle. In this context, the assumption is that something in my current lifestyle is restricting my body from healing. Therefore, I need to make some kind of change to kick-start the recovery process. In the case of my shoulder, I realized I wasn't sitting with good posture at work. This was putting stress on certain tissues that could have done without it. I was also sleeping poorly, so I had to introduce pillows to prop up my arm at night and refrain from certain gym routines that seemed to aggravate the shoulder.

Making lifestyle changes might be as simple as not sitting for so long each day, to as consequential as changing your job in order to allow an injury to heal. I met a man who was forced to leave his job in the fire service because of a chronic case of tennis elbow which had been slowly getting worse for more than 10 years. Only then did he start to get better.

If you have tried to fix an injury through targeted exercise and lifestyle changes, yet it is showing no sign of improvement, I would then move on to the third stage of the plan, which is to see if medication helps. I am very averse to taking pain pills. However, there are some instances when they can be useful, to an extent. Sometimes, a short course of medication can provide a window of opportunity for the other two methods to start to take effect. If pain prevents the exercise, which may be possible when a painkiller is taken, a short course might be a good idea. I would always then have the goal of reducing the dose of those painkillers as quickly as possible. In the case of my shoulder,

I did have a period of time where I would take an ibuprofen tablet at night to allow me to sleep a little better. Taking the pill in that case was the lesser of two evils.

If all of the above fails, then (and only then) should the fourth option be considered: surgery. I fundamentally believe that the body has an incredible healing power housed within. Any time we cut the body open and mess with its inherent structures, I believe we interrupt its natural healing ability. However, there are times when surgery is required and undoubtedly examples of it leading to a miraculous recovery. I would always approach the idea of surgery with extreme caution. It should never be seen as a quick and easy fix, and the long-term consequences of surgery should not be minimized. In my case, I did at one time see a specialist for a second opinion on my shoulder. She offered me surgery, but, to her credit, recommended I continue with rehab for at least another month or two. By the grace of fate, this seemed somehow to kick my shoulder into action, and I never needed to go back to her—something I am grateful for every day!

This set of principles helps me to guide my patients through a set of options in treating their injuries. I almost always start at the top and work my way down. Thankfully, the vast majority of people can get better by implementing the first and second stages alone.

Now, in the following pages of this book, we're going to talk about specific areas of the body, one by one. My hope is that in each chapter, you'll learn something useful that you can apply to your own life or routine, in order to improve your health, fitness and longevity. Let's get started with the head, neck and shoulders.

Part Two

HEAD, NECK AND SHOULDERS

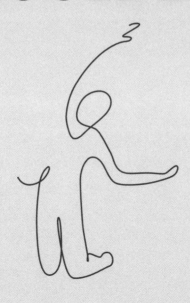

Introduction

In this chapter, I'm going to share my stories, expert information and best guidance for problems involving the head, neck and shoulders. In my clinic, I regularly help people not just with painful necks and shoulders, but with their headaches as well. These problems are often linked. For example, it's common to find that when a client's neck pain is treated, their headaches also disappear.

In the pages that follow, you'll find out about the best sleeping positions, the best time to get a massage, how to ease a stiff neck, the truth about your posture and much more. The problems we talk about in this chapter are incredibly common. If you're suffering with one of these issues, don't panic! You're certainly not alone.

Let's start by talking about the normal function of the neck—and how you can restore yours.

The Six Key Movements
of the Neck

The human neck is a wonderful and intricate invention. Made up of seven cervical vertebrae, as many discs and a network of nerves and blood vessels, it is no wonder we are always taught to be careful with our necks during sport and physical activity.

Even if you were to take good care of your neck throughout your younger years, you would not be guaranteed a healthy neck in the latter half of your life. Many people suffer with age-related deterioration to the facet joints and discs that make up the moving parts of the neck. If left unchecked, these normal aging changes can lead to abnormal levels of pain and stiffness. Thankfully, even for the stiffest of necks, there is often a lot that can be done to help tackle the problem.

To provide a solution, the first thing to understand is what a normal pattern of neck movement looks like. Our necks have six "pure" movements available: flexion, extension, side flexion to the left and right, and rotation to the left and right. These movements are depicted opposite.

As we age, all six of these movements (but especially extension and rotation) can become restricted. The simplest way to regain movement of your neck is to practice each of the movements gently and repeatedly over a period of time. The positions only need to be held for a couple of moments and it's not necessary to push into uncomfortable ranges of motion. As a good place to start, I recommend performing movements for the stiffer areas of your neck within a comfortable range, about 10 times in a row, about three times per day.

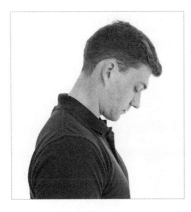

Flexion: Gently tilt your head forward.

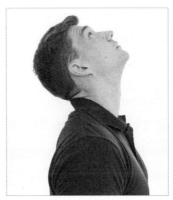

Extension: Gently tilt your head backward.

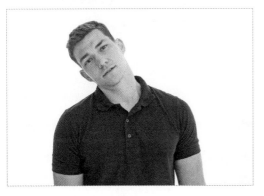

Right side flexion: Gently tilt your head downward toward your right shoulder.

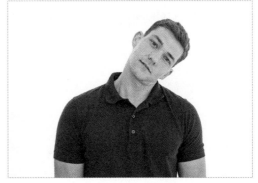

Left side flexion: Gently tilt your head downward toward your left shoulder.

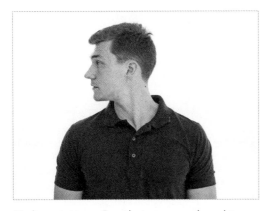

Right rotation: Gently turn your head to the right.

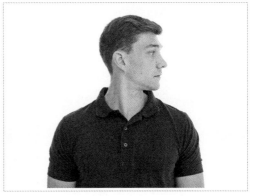

Left rotation: Gently turn your head to the left.

It is incredible how much difference such a simple practice can make to neck mobility. If you have noticed that you have trouble looking up at things, or you notice stiffness when turning your head while driving, you might be a good candidate for this exercise.

I would encourage you to stick to the pure neck movements only when practising. I often see people trying to combine these movements with rolling the neck from one ear to the other behind the shoulders, for example. These movements are not necessary to free up the neck and may actually make pain worse by pinching on the facet joints.

There are other exercises to improve neck mobility in the following pages, too. First, however, let's talk about the normal movements of the shoulder joint.

The Four
Most Important Shoulder
Movements

The shoulder is one of the most complex joints in the whole body, not necessarily in structure but in function. It is a ball-and-socket joint, and it has more freedom of movement than any other joint in the body. But with this level of mobility comes a burden: if the control we have over our shoulder movement is not optimal, problems very quickly appear. Shoulder problems can also be notoriously painful. Indeed, the shoulder is probably my least favorite part of the body to treat in the clients who come to see me at my practice, partly due to its complexity.

One way to prevent the development of many common shoulder problems is to ensure your shoulders are moving optimally for as much of your life as possible. We want to maintain both the mobility and control of our shoulder joints. The first step to achieving this is to understand a bit more about how a normal shoulder joint moves. There are many movements available to the shoulder joint; however, there are four that are commonly affected by the process of aging: flexion, abduction and internal and external rotation. These can all be seen on page 48.

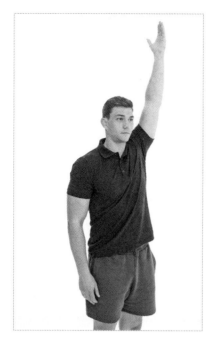

Shoulder flexion

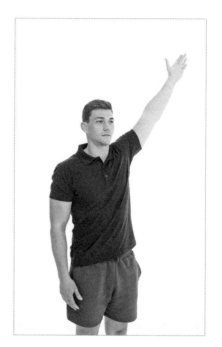

Shoulder abduction

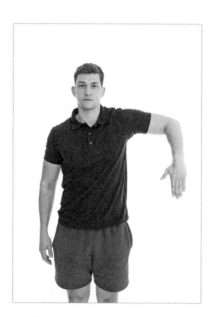

Shoulder internal rotation

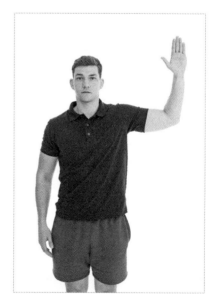

Shoulder external rotation

Just as with the neck, practising these movements in their purest form regularly can help a stiff shoulder to regain its movement. However, giving yourself a literal "helping hand" can also be greatly beneficial when it comes to restoring mobility. By using the opposite hand to assist the stiffer side, it's possible to regain lost movement over time. This is a rehabilitation technique I share with many of my clients whose stiff shoulders are contributing to their symptoms. It is possible to use the opposite hand alone, or to use a tool (like a walking stick) to assist the movement further. To illustrate this technique in action, look at the pictures below and on page 50.

With the hand of your stiff shoulder (below, that's my right shoulder) leading the movement, use your other hand to move the stick in each direction repetitively, stopping at the point of natural resistance.

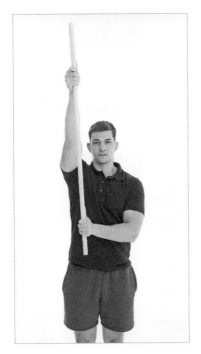
Shoulder flexion with stick

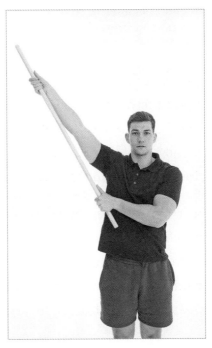
Shoulder abduction with stick

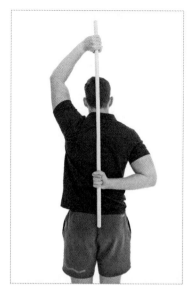
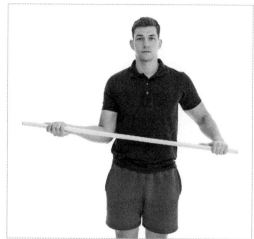

Shoulder internal
rotation with stick

Shoulder external rotation with stick

For all of these exercises, I tell my clients to focus on the movement that seems stiffest and then repeat a tiny, rhythmical "bounce" (one second in, one second out), moving just an inch or so at the very end of the natural range. This should not be a painful motion. The movement should come to an end just as you reach the edges of stiffness, retreating back into a comfortable range each time.

This tiny but repeated movement has the potential to improve natural range of motion and restore mobility when worked over a period of time. As with many of the exercises in this book, the frequency (i.e. how often you come back to the exercise) matters more than how much you do in one go. It is almost always better to do these exercises for one minute, three times a day, than it is to do them for three minutes all in one go.

How to Ensure
Lifelong Shoulder Health

Throughout most of our lives, our arms hang by our sides or are only ever slightly in front of us. Looking down at my posture right now as I type this sentence, my upper arm is flexed about 20 degrees in front of my body. For most people, this is exactly how their arms are positioned almost all day. Except for the occasional reach for something overhead, in the modern world our arms barely leave our sides.

Over time, this way of life leads to problems with the shoulder joints. Confined to our sides all day, the shoulder is almost never taken through its full range of motion. There is a great deal of truth to the saying "if you don't use it, you lose it," and this rings true with our shoulder range of motion.

To test this, try lifting your arms directly above your head. We should have 180 degrees of shoulder flexion, meaning we should all have the ability to point our arms vertically in the air. The sad truth is most of us lose the ability to do this somewhere along the way. These changes do not happen suddenly; they are the product of years of disuse in certain ranges of motion. The problem with this loss of motion at the shoulder joint is that a stiff shoulder is more likely to suffer arthritis, injury and problems with the rotator cuff. These problems can lead to pain and disability at any age, but more commonly in people over the age of fifty.

For many, regaining range of motion at the shoulder is possible, provided you know how to do so safely. Other than using the exercises in the previous chapter, I have found two great ways to regain shoulder flexion, one of which is simple and the other advanced. The simple way is by standing in a doorframe and reaching overhead until your hand or wrist can touch the doorframe above you; this is assisted flexion. Slowly move your body forward until your shoulder is gently pushed into flexion (*see right*). The end position should feel like a comfortable stretch (and should not be painful). Hold this position for 20 to 30 seconds, then change sides. If you're not tall enough to reach a doorframe, you can try the self-assisted flexion exercise on page 81.

The second technique is advanced and is probably out of the question for the majority of over-fifties. However, I appreciate there are a range of abilities in my audience, so this exercise is for the stronger and more able individuals. It requires ample strength in the upper body, including the hands, and access to a safe pull-up bar (improvised kit is NOT advised). If you are a regular gym-goer and can support your body weight with your grip, this exercise might be suitable for you. This exercise is called the dead hang, and involves hanging from a pull-up bar while trying to allow your shoulders to relax as gravity pulls your body weight down toward the floor (*see right*). Just hanging for half a minute is enough to feel a significant improvement in shoulder stiffness for many people, and there is some evidence to show this position has the potential to "decompress" the spine, too.

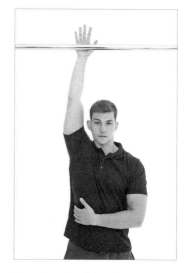

Regain shoulder flexion: Start by raising your arm above your head. Rest the palm of your hand on the doorframe. Gently move your body forward until you feel a stretch in your shoulder. Hold this stretch for 20 to 30 seconds.

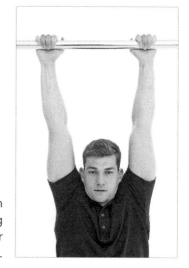

The 'dead hang': Tightly grasp the pull-up bar with both hands. Slowly transfer your weight off your feet, relying on your hands to support your body weight. Allow your shoulders to relax away from your body as you hang.

Could Your Neck Be Giving You Headaches?

Headaches are an incredibly common problem, and 95 percent of people will suffer from a headache at some point in their lives. In fact, on any given day, 11 percent of men and 22 percent of women will be suffering from a headache.[1] For some, this pain can be daily and extremely debilitating.

For those who do suffer with frequent headaches, my first thought would be to try to help them identify the underlying cause of these. We would start by asking them to try to explain the characteristics of their headache.

Is it like a tight band around the head? Does it only affect the back of the head, or the whole head? Does it feel like a pulsating pain behind the eyes? Or is it more of a continuous ache? All of these questions can help to pinpoint the root cause of a headache (which is paramount to treating it).

Now, not many people know this, but many headaches in adults are caused by problems in the neck. We call this type of problem "cervicogenic headaches."

Have you ever suffered from a stiff neck with pain radiating up into the back of your head? If you have, you'll know just how unpleasant a headache like this can be. Some of my clients tell me a headache like this is much worse than the neck pain associated with it.

The interesting thing is that it is also possible to suffer from cervicogenic headaches without feeling any neck pain whatsoever. This can make it very hard to tell whether the neck is responsible—or if the culprit is something else entirely.

Here are a few clues which can help you identify a neck-related headache:

- You might feel the headache at the back of the head, on one or both sides, or it could be round the sides of the head, too. Less common is pain behind the eyes or across the forehead.

- Your headache might get worse when you turn your head, when you drive or turn to speak to someone, for example.

- The headache will usually be more like a dull ache than a sharp pain.

- You might also have some neck pain, although neck pain is not a prerequisite for cervicogenic headaches.

The cause behind these neck-related headaches is usually the fact that either the muscles in the neck are too tight or the joints aren't moving quite as well as they should be. We call these "mechanical" issues and they can be caused by a number of differing factors. Arthritis, muscle strains and whiplash can all cause cervicogenic headaches, too.

Be sure to get any new persistent headache assessed by your doctor first, but here are some top tips to help with this problem at home:

- **Check for other causes:** If you aren't sure whether it is indeed your neck that is causing your headaches, it is worth ruling out other potential causes first. Dehydration, hormonal problems and vitamin deficiencies can all cause headaches. It's worth getting a thorough examination (possibly including blood tests) before you go any further.

- **Keep your neck mobile:** The stiffer it gets, the worse the headache. Moving your neck might initially make the pain a little worse, but it should get better in the long run with some gentle movement within a comfortable range.

- **Use heat treatment on your neck:** Applying a warm compress to the back of your neck for 15 minutes at a time (be sure to protect the skin) can help to ease tight muscles and loosen stiff joints. Even if the pain is only in the head, this will often still help!

- **Try the towel-assisted rotation exercise:** Described on pages 57–59, this exercise can help with pain relief and to restore the range of motion in your neck, provided it's safe for you to do so.

- **Check your sleeping position, as it's important:** If lying on your side, your neck and head should be in line with your shoulders, as if you were upright. Try to experiment with an extra pillow, or take one away if you currently use more than one, to see if that improves matters. Sometimes, getting a new pillow might be a good idea. If you sleep on your back, use a supportive pillow and a rolled towel to ensure the head and neck are supported in the position shown below.

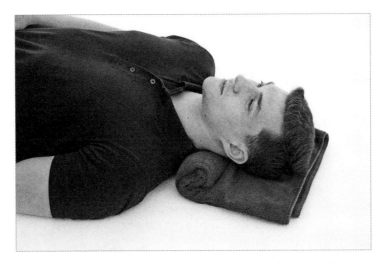

This resting position is ideal for maintaining the natural curve in your neck.

- **Watch your posture:** By gently pulling your shoulder blades back and down when you sit (rather than rounding your shoulders) you can often relieve some of the stress in tired neck muscles and improve your headaches as a result. Try to imagine your lower back, mid back, shoulders and head stacked atop one another and balancing there when you're sitting still. Far more important than sitting in the "correct" posture (*see also page 64*) is not spending too long in any one posture. Try to get up and move or change positions regularly.

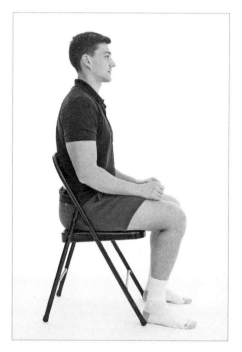

Although no posture is 'perfect', good sitting posture can be maintained by imagining everything 'stacked' on top of each other when sitting.

Relieve Neck Pain and Stiffness with One Exercise!

One of the most common questions I get asked by the people who come to see me in my clinic is: "How do I get rid of this stiff neck?"

A stiff neck often starts slowly, creeping in gradually over the course of several days. It can also start rapidly, sometimes being a nasty surprise to wake up with one day.

Luckily, there is a gentle approach that can usually help with neck pain and stiffness. It works especially well for people over fifty, as the root cause of their neck pain is often something we call a "facet joint dysfunction." That's a fancy term for a situation where the joints in the neck aren't quite moving as they should.

There are seven bones in your neck and the way they work is quite intricate. They all move in a synchronized way, articulating with one another via seven joints on each side of the neck, powered by the surrounding muscles.

If, for some reason, one of the 14 joints becomes stiff or the muscles that support movement become imbalanced, a facet joint dysfunction can occur. I like to picture a facet joint dysfunction as a poorly fitted cupboard door, with the hinging mechanism not properly working. This makes it difficult to use the joint as it was designed and can make the neck seem stiff and painful.

Another possible issue is a muscle spasm, which can arise from the same cause. If there is a problem with movement, the body senses a problem and goes on red alert. The way your body then acts to "protect" you from harm is to tighten up and send the muscles into spasm as a safety mechanism. The spasm is a signal from the body that says, "Don't move, it's not safe!" On the surface, this might seem like a stupid response but it's actually very clever. Your brain isn't able to differentiate between a genuine and a false risk of harm. It can't be sure you aren't about to suffer an injury. Therefore, in order to prevent you from suffering a serious injury, it takes away the risk by restricting your movement.

So, if you haven't damaged anything but your neck is still stiff and sore, how are we supposed to fix it?

The answer is that we have to show the body it's safe to move again, and the towel-assisted rotation exercise below and opposite will help you do exactly that.

This exercise is a type of mobilization that uses an external force (the towel) to help the stiff facet joints to move as they were designed to do, thus returning full range of motion and easing stiffness. This exercise also helps to relieve the symptoms of a muscle spasm by "calming" the nervous system in the affected area, allowing more freedom of movement and less pain.

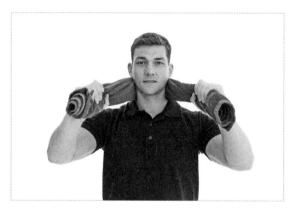

1. Start by rolling a hand towel lengthways into a band. Place the band around the back of your neck, just at the point where the head meets the neck. Pull firmly forward adding tension to the towel.

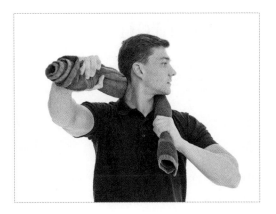

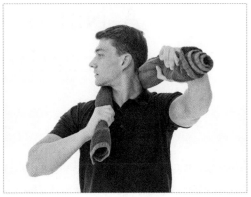

2. Keeping the tension on the towel throughout, turn your head to the left, and as you do so, pull forward with your right hand. You might find that you are able to turn your head further than you normally can.

3. Keep the tension on the band as you return to the centre. Then repeat, turning to the right but pulling forward with your left hand. Repeat 10 times in each direction, several times a day.

A Natural Approach to Treating Migraines

Throughout my childhood, there would sometimes be whole days, even weeks, where my mother couldn't get out of bed. She could barely open her eyes or speak during these episodes. I didn't fully understand it at the time: why was she behaving so strangely? It wasn't until I was old enough to understand that she told me that these terrible times were caused by migraines.

Anyone who's suffered with a migraine so fierce that they want to do nothing other than lock themselves in their closet will be able to tell you how debilitating they can be. Contrary to what many people believe, a true migraine is not the same as a simple headache.

There are several medications available that are designed to treat migraines and, for many people, these are sufficient to reduce the frequency or intensity of the suffering. But for a good number, these medications don't solve the underlying cause.

What is often missed is an imbalance in the body somewhere, causing these chronic migraines. Your migraines could actually be caused by a deficiency in certain vitamins and minerals, or an intolerance to a common food in your diet.

My initial advice to anyone coming to me with migraines is to first get the levels of vitamins and minerals in their blood tested. You can find relatively inexpensive vitamin and mineral blood tests online, or ask your doctor for one.

Magnesium, vitamin B and coenzyme Q10 supplements have been shown to help migraines in some promising clinical trials.[2] This book is all about finding natural ways to treat even the most stubborn issues; if you're fed up with taking medication for your migraines this may be something you want to read more about and discuss with your doctor to see if it is suitable for you.

Something you should bear in mind is that migraines have been linked consistently with hormonal fluctuations throughout a woman's life. We all know about menopause, and speaking to your doctor about balancing your hormones if they are running amok can often go a long way to fixing the issue at its root cause.

Failing that, the thing that worked for my mother was an elimination diet. She slowly cut out various suspect foods from her diet until she found two clear triggers for her awful migraines: cocoa and coffee. Unfortunately, her body didn't care that these were her favorite treats. However, she wouldn't hesitate to say that cutting these foods from her diet was worth the return to normality, without persistent 72-hour-long migraines.

Migraines, just like headaches, can also be triggered by a problem with the neck. Stiffness in the facet joints (particularly in the upper cervical spine) can lead to migraines if left unchecked, as can tightness in the neck muscles. I have had many patients who first notice neck stiffness as a warning sign before a severe migraine.

Ultimately, it is important for migraine sufferers to recognize that there are many potential triggers for migraines. It may be that you can tolerate one isolated trigger, but when two or more are combined, a fierce migraine begins. Identify your triggers and do your best to avoid them where you can.

Why You Need More Than Massage to Fix Your Neck Pain

One thing that took me a long time to understand when it comes to pain is the fact that the painful area isn't always the source of the problem.

When I first started my career as a physiotherapist, people would come to see me about their neck pain and point to their neck saying, "This is where it hurts." Diligently, I would provide treatment and exercises, all targeted at the painful area. For some, I'd get good results. However, for many, they would only get temporary relief. They'd tell me how the exercises would work . . . *for about five minutes*. Then it'd be back to square one.

I couldn't understand how I wasn't making progress with these people in my first year of practice. It wasn't until another year or so that I realized I wasn't treating the problem at all. I was simply masking the surface-level problem. My methods back then were on a par with painkillers—concealing the symptoms without resolving the underlying cause.

A paradigm-shifting moment came for me when I started to address not just the symptoms but the driving force behind the neck complaint. For many people, the neck pain was only a symptom. The underlying cause was hiding somewhere else entirely.

The truth is, for many people who suffer from neck pain when sitting, driving or working, there will be a group of muscles that are working far too hard. This tends to be the painful region. Why are these muscles working too hard? The reason is because there is usually another group of muscles somewhere in the vicinity *which are not working hard enough*. These lazy muscles aren't doing their job properly, so the stronger muscles in the neck decide to take over. They think, "If those lazy muscles aren't doing their job, I guess I'm going to have to pick up the slack!"

And that's where the problem starts. These stronger, overworked muscles are now doing two jobs instead of the one job they were designed for. It's no wonder they start to complain after a while. And when a muscle complains, its way of doing so is by giving you pain!

So, let's bring it back to the treatment room. If I were to massage your tight, tired muscles—the ones that are doing all the work—it might make them feel good for a while. But as soon as you start to move again, they still have to pick up the slack from the other muscles that have effectively "switched off."

This means that we need to take a different approach to treating neck pain. We can't just rub the painful area and expect the pain not to come back. How easy life would be if that were true!

What we need to do instead is to encourage the lazy muscles in our neck and upper body to start working a bit harder, to begin doing their job again, rather than passing the buck to the all-too-eager muscles that end up overworked and in pain.

The next few sections of this book are dedicated to giving you a few strategies for doing just that. Sure, massage is useful alongside the techniques on the following pages, but never rely on massage alone to get that neck better. Instead, let's have a look at some more effective strategies.

The Truth about Posture

When a physiotherapist starts to talk about neck pain, everyone expects that the next line to come out of their mouth will be something along the lines of: " . . . and you need to watch your posture!" It's become widely expected that you'll get some kind of postural advice in every physiotherapy session. Many of my clients glumly admit to me that they have "poor posture," even before I've assessed them.

But what exactly is poor posture?

Is poor posture just slouching? Or is there more to it than that?

My definition of "poor posture" is simply a position that is suboptimal for the performance of a given task, whether that be sitting, standing or walking. This means that posture must always be assessed in the context of the task at hand.

To make matters more complicated, we are all built differently. Some of us have long legs and a short body, while others have long spines or even a leg-length difference. This means *your* so-called "perfect posture" is going to be completely different to that of your neighbor for any given task.

All of this being said, there are some general rules to follow that still apply to all. It makes sense to sit and stand in a way that puts the least stress on our joints and muscles. By following a set of principles that apply to almost all of us, we can minimize stress and strain on the body over time.

One of the ways we can do this is by assuming the position that minimizes the strain put on the body by gravity. The detrimental effects of gravity are minimized when the vertebrae making up the spine are "stacked" on top of one another. If we ignore this principle, we can get into trouble. If we sit or stand in a way that positions the head in front of the shoulders, gravity is going to act to pull the head downward, with the muscles at the back of our neck being put under immense strain to resist this. If our shoulders are rounded, the curvature of the spine is exaggerated and gravity acts more harshly on the spinal joints. These are just two examples of how subtle changes to posture can lead to an increase in mechanical stress over time.

Now that almost all of us use computers, laptops, tablets and phones every day, a huge proportion of our day is spent looking at the gadget in our hand or on our laps. The use of these gadgets encourages us to poke our chins forward as we strain to see small print, and to round our shoulders as we use our hands to type. These subtle postural changes take our neck and shoulders out of "alignment," putting undue stress on weaker muscles. It's no wonder that people who work in office jobs, or spend a lot of time on social media, are far more likely to suffer neck pain than their more active counterparts.

When we get up after a prolonged laptop session, the muscles that became shortened during our time spent sitting don't automatically return to their normal length. This means we tend to remain in this new, poor posture long after the gadget is put down.

The first step to correcting this issue is simply to be aware that it is happening. Once you're aware of it, you can ask yourself, "Are my shoulders tipped forward and rounded? Is my chin poking forward?"

Sometimes, my clients only realize their posture has become a problem when they happen to catch a sideways glance of themselves in the reflection of a shop window. Thankfully, if you have noticed your posture has slipped, there are subtle yet effective changes you can make to take the pressure off these key areas again.

There are two great "cues" you can use to help you do this. One cue is to imagine your sternum (the hard bone that sits in the middle of your chest) is a full glass of water.

When you walk around with your shoulders rounded, your sternum tends to be tilted forward, spilling water from this imaginary glass down your front.

Now, to stop the spillage: slightly pull your shoulders back and push your chest out a little. Notice how your sternum tilts back—it should be perfectly upright now, and the water will stay in the glass. Use this visualization whenever you get up after sitting at a laptop or on the phone for any length of time.

To improve your posture while walking, there is another great visualization I commonly teach my clients. Imagine a piece of string attached to the top of your head. Picture what would happen if a magical force from above pulled on the string to make you as tall as possible. You'd feel yourself grow an inch, your chest would rise and your shoulders would move backward slightly. For most people, this happens to be an excellent posture to maintain while walking, taking pressure off the neck and mid back. These slight tweaks can offer an effective solution to pain in these areas.

There is another simple solution that can help to fix poor posture when walking— consciously choosing your gaze.

Most people walk around with their eyes looking down at the floor. This is especially the case in more senior individuals who may feel their balance is no longer what it was. Their eyes tend to drift toward the floor to avoid tripping on uneven ground. However, this presents a problem. Their head tends to follow their gaze, making it more likely to move in front of the shoulders. This brings the center of gravity forward, potentially increasing the chance of a forward fall by placing the individual off balance.

The solution to this problem? Fix your gaze at the floor, but no less than 4.5m (15ft) ahead. For most people, 4.5m (15ft) ahead is far enough to force them to lift their eyes and head, but not so far as to make it impossible to see the ground ahead. This is a fantastic compromise, allowing the safety that watching the ground can bring, without the detriment to balance.

Re-engage Those Lazy Muscles

In the previous section, we spoke about how to become more aware of what "good posture" is and how to avoid spending too much time in suboptimal postures. That simple awareness alone will go a long way toward taking strain and tension away from your neck and shoulders.

However, there is still a problem for most people. Due to a lifetime of poor postural habits, there are certain muscles that remain tight and overused, while others remain weak and underused. These weak muscles are essentially "lazy"; they have shrugged their workload onto their bigger, stronger cousins so that they can take to the back seat and enjoy a free ride.

To complete the puzzle and solve poor posture, we still need to work on re-engaging the muscles around the neck and shoulders that have effectively "switched off." What we're going to do in this chapter is learn exactly how to kick-start these commonly lazy muscles and have them pick up the slack again.

The muscles we are going to work on strengthening sit between your shoulder blades and are called the rhomboids. They are responsible for keeping your shoulders in good alignment when you perform delicate tasks that involve using your arms (such as using a mouse or keyboard).

You'll need a light resistance band for the following exercise. You can buy these very cheaply online or from your local sports store. You won't need much resistance to start off with, so get the thinnest band you can find to practice with first.

Once you've got your resistance band, you're going to do the following:

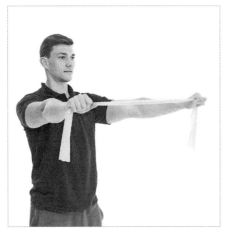 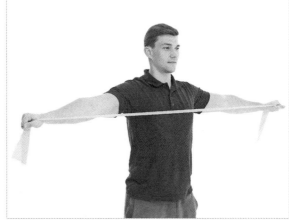

1. Hold the band in both hands with your palms facing down, with some slack in the band between your hands. Raise your arms straight up in front of you so that they come up to chest level. Don't let your shoulders 'shrug' up toward your ears; keep them relaxed and low.

2. Keeping your shoulders relaxed and low, pull the band apart as far as you possibly can, by engaging the muscles between your shoulder blades. Once you've pulled the band right across your chest, make every effort to squeeze your shoulder blades together once more, as if you're trying to pinch a pencil between them. Hold this position for three to five seconds, then slowly let the band return to the start position in front of your chest.

Repeat this resistance band pull-apart exercise until you get a slight working ache between your shoulder blades, or until you can't stop your shoulders from shrugging up toward your ears—whichever comes first.

My Favorite Exercise for Upper-Body Mobility

When I started my career in the NHS, I used to suffer from pain in the thoracic spine (mid back) that got worse as the working day went on. The irony of a young physio suffering from posture-related pain was not lost on me, so I kept quiet—but some days I would have to lie on the treatment couch between patients just to find relief. I knew the problem was, in part, because I was forced to sit on a little stool with wheels at a miniature school-like desk to write my clinical notes. At the time, our notes were still written with pen and paper, meaning I was forced into a strange posture over my little desk for several hours a day.

Thoracic pain is common, and much of the time it is caused by suboptimal posture. Sitting in a rounded posture (like many of us do) leads to a reduction in available range of motion at the thoracic spine, particularly in a movement called extension. Extension is the direction of movement involved in leaning back. A reduced range of extension in the thoracic spine has been associated with thoracic pain.[3] Sitting at my poorly positioned desk on my poorly positioned stool was the cause of my rounded back, which then caused my thoracic pain.

I know I am not the only one who suffers with this issue. My patients tell me about thoracic pain regularly. Luckily, I found an exercise that worked well for me and works well for my patients, too. This exercise is designed to restore lost thoracic extension and, in addition to relieving many cases of mid-back pain, it can take pressure off the shoulders and lower back, too.

Below you can see how to perform this thoracic extension exercise. Technique is very important, with a particular focus on not rounding the lower back but keeping it flat. The movement should occur at the mid back, and movement here may be extremely limited at first. It is also important to state that it took me a long time and many repetitions of doing this exercise to restore the lost mobility in my thoracic spine, so do not expect miracles from the first few days of practice!

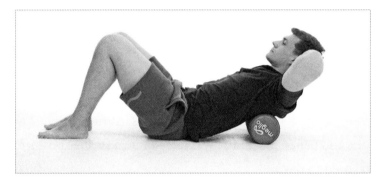

1. Place a foam roller on a mat and position it so that it lies horizontally across your back, at about the level of your shoulder blades. Support your head in your hands to prevent neck pain.

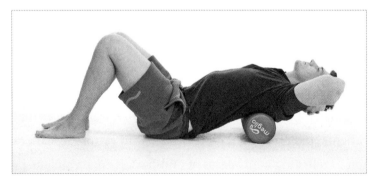

2. Without arching your lower back, slowly lean back over the foam roller. Stop at the point of stiffness, then return to the starting position.

The Tiny Neck Muscles
That Can Prevent Arthritis

The human neck is an incredible example of nature's architecture at its finest. One of the most complex areas of the human body, the neck houses intricate bony structures, branches and bundles of nerves and muscles that work both independently and together as a unit. As mentioned earlier, our necks tend to feel better if we sit and stand in a position where all the structures within the neck are properly "stacked" on top of each other.

Think of it like a game of Jenga: if you stack the blocks correctly, the tower is stable. However, if you stack them in a rush, with some of the little wooden blocks askew, your tower is no longer as stable and is, instead, prone to stress and strain. Our necks are no different. Stacked correctly, we can minimize the stress put on the tiny joints in the neck.

Unlike Jenga, we can't add or subtract the bones in our neck. However, we can change the pulling force on these bones by asking certain muscles to do the jobs they were designed for.

One of the reasons we want to limit undue stress and strain on our intricate neck joints is because this helps to prevent arthritis. "Arthritis" is a term used to describe the (natural or accelerated) wearing down of the cartilage within our joints, and I'll refer to it many times throughout the course of this book.

If you've been told that you already have some arthritis in your neck, this need not always be cause for concern. I find the exercises I use to help people prevent arthritis are often the exact same ones I might use to treat it, so this chapter can still help.

A group of tiny muscles is located within your neck, under your chin. They are collectively referred to as the deep neck flexors. They are given the daunting task of supporting your head when you sit, walk and move. In order to support the weight of the head (which is enormous in comparison to the size of these tiny muscles), it is vital that these muscles are strong and durable enough to do their job well, no matter how small they might be.

So, how do we know if these tiny muscles are working properly?

If you find that the back of your neck aches after you've been driving any distance, or you've noticed that your chin pokes forward when you sit or walk, it's likely that the deep neck flexors aren't doing their job very well at all. You might also notice a "compressed" feeling at the back of your neck, as if something is being trapped or crushed there. That feeling may be the weight of your head putting strain on the neck joints, which is something that should be prevented by the deep neck flexors. If left untreated, this continuous pressure can cause problems later down the line. But don't worry—this is solvable.

The exercise that follows is a fantastic way to resolve this "crushing" sensation at the back of the neck, helping with neck pain, headaches and stiffness. Called the chin tuck, it's a very subtle exercise that doesn't require much effort, just plenty of regularity. Lots of my patients find that they can quite happily get on with this exercise in front of the TV or in the car.

Here's how you can find the muscles we want to activate: from a sitting position, keep your eyes level and pull your chin in, as if to make a double chin. The muscles you can feel working are the ones we are going to target.

I usually recommend most people try to dedicate at least 10 minutes a day, split evenly into smaller chunks of time, to practising this exercise. It is perfect for most people who are suffering from neck pain, or those who would like to take out an insurance policy against neck arthritis in the future. Repeat the movement for several minutes whenever sitting still for any length of time.

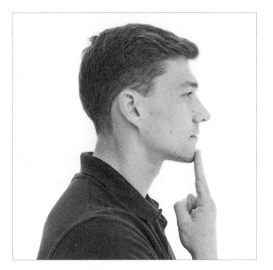

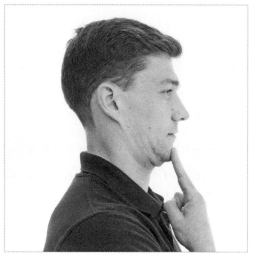

1. Start by sitting upright somewhere comfortable with your eyes looking straight ahead.

2. Gently pull your chin in as if you're trying to make a subtle double chin. Keep your eyes gazing straight ahead and don't let your nose move toward the floor as you do this. Hold this position for five seconds, then relax to your normal position.

Counter the Effects of Sitting

It isn't just the neck that gets stiff from sitting. There is another part of the body that suffers, even though it tends not to complain quite so much. This area is the mid back, or thoracic spine.

The surprising truth is that many people don't know that this area of their body has a problem. But just because there isn't any pain there, that doesn't mean it isn't incredibly stiff. And stiffness in the thoracic spine is a big problem for the rest of the body.

First, the mid back is the region of the spine that allows you to twist. There isn't very much rotation available at your lower back, so even though you may feel like you're rotating at the lower back when you turn your torso, 90 percent of that movement is coming from the middle section of your spine. When the thoracic spine loses the ability to rotate, which area of the body do you think is required to pick up the slack? That's right, the lower back. The problem is the lower back is now being asked to do a job it wasn't designed to do, causing increased stress in this area. This is why problems with the thoracic spine can contribute to lumbar spine (lower-back) pain.

Second, there is another vital movement of the mid back, called extension (otherwise known as leaning back). Being able to extend from the thoracic spine allows us to walk and stand without putting too much pressure on other areas of the body. However, the vast majority of people have completely lost the ability to extend through the thoracic spine. This is most common in desk workers, or people who sit a lot. Being in a seated position increases the curvature in your thoracic spine, placing you in a flexed-forward position. Being flexed forward is the opposite of extension or leaning back, so if we spend our days locked in flexion, when we come to extend the thoracic spine, it is common to find we have lost the ability to perform this movement at all.

The old saying is absolutely true: if you don't use it, you lose it!

When we lose the ability to extend freely at the thoracic spine, other areas need to pick up the slack—and it tends to be the neck that draws the short straw. This is why much neck pain can actually be attributed to a stiff mid back, rather than a problem with the neck itself.

So, how can your mid back become so stiff all of a sudden?

The real truth is . . . the process is not very sudden at all! The mid back becomes stiff and restricted over a period of years and the sitting position tends to be responsible for much of this disastrous loss of movement.

Luckily, all is not lost, even if you've spent half your life working an office job. Even if you're stiff, you can work to regain some of that lost movement.

So, we need to find a way to improve the two movements most people have lost: thoracic rotation and extension.

The two-minute seated-rotation routine that follows will help many with thoracic back pain, as well as those who suffer from neck pain and stiffness. I would recommend this routine be done after sitting or driving for any distance, or just whenever there is a sensation of stiffness in the thoracic spine.

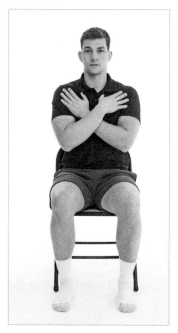 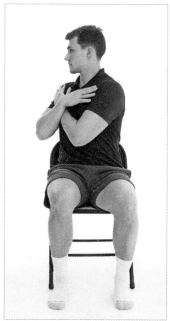 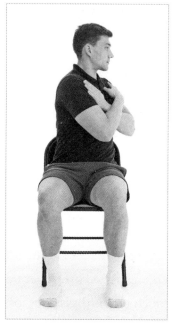

1. Start by sitting in a chair with arms crossed over your chest.

2. Slowly and carefully, turn your upper body to the right.

3. Then, still moving slowly and carefully, turn to the left. Rotate right and left 10 times in a row, three times per day.

Get Relief from a Frozen Shoulder

The dreaded frozen shoulder: intense pain, sleep disturbance and an inability to use one arm for an extended period of time, due to months of debilitating stiffness. The worst part is, there is usually no obvious trigger for the problem. It's no wonder my patients groan when they get this diagnosis.

If you've been diagnosed with a frozen shoulder, or suspect you might have one, it's important to understand this condition a little better before attempting to treat it.

Frozen shoulder is a problem the medical world doesn't yet fully understand. Scientists have not yet identified an absolute trigger for what causes it,[4] but we know there are some risk factors that make frozen shoulder more likely (such as being female, diabetic or having thyroid problems[5]).

A frozen shoulder starts with intense pain in the shoulder. Usually, the pain is reported as being just below the shoulder joint, leading some people to think they have an issue with the arm as opposed to the joint. The pain can be incredibly severe, often reaching a crescendo in one to three months. After that, the pain usually reduces, while profound stiffness takes its place. And as quickly and mysteriously as frozen shoulder started, it will eventually disappear on its own as well.

If you're suffering at the moment from a frozen shoulder, it's important to know that you're not alone: around 3 percent of the population will go through this at some point in their lifetime.[3] It is also vital that you keep in mind that this problem will eventually get better; although that often feels like cold comfort when it is keeping you awake night after night.

The shoulder pendulum exercise that follows can also be an effective pain-reliever. It produces an effect called "traction" on the shoulder joint, which basically means gently and safely pulling the shoulder joint apart to create a nice "gap" in the joint. This allows more lubricating synovial fluid into the joint, which reduces some of the constricting pressure in the shoulder. I like to think of synovial fluid as the body's very own version of WD-40, improving movement and reducing stiffness.

For this exercise, all you'll need is a small weight or dumbbell to hold. Alternatively, you could use a rucksack or sturdy bag and fill it with some books. Only persist with this exercise if it feels as though it relieves your pain. It should not be painful and should feel better afterward. The movement should be small and controlled.

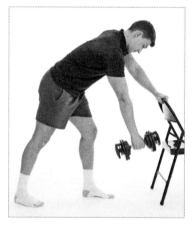

1. Start by holding a weight in your hand on the affected side. For support, place your other hand on a chair or worktop. Lean forward so that your affected shoulder is hanging down.

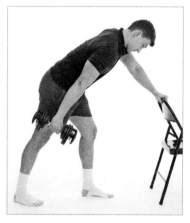

2. Slowly start to swing the weight like a pendulum, forward and back. As you do this, try to let gravity do the work and let your shoulder relax as much as you can. Continue for 30 seconds, two to three times a day.

If your frozen shoulder is disturbing your sleep and getting in the way of your daily routine, it might be worth speaking to your doctor about pain relief. Often, a steroid injection can be considered to reduce the severe pain associated with the condition. I don't often recommend steroid injections to my clients (due to the risks associated) but if your shoulder is stopping you from sleeping, this kind of treatment might be worth considering.

Defrost Your Frozen Shoulder

If you're suffering from a true frozen shoulder, the initial excruciating pain should pass within a few months. However, what you will be left with is a shoulder that really doesn't want to move.

This is what gives a frozen shoulder its name. I've had clients whose arms become literally pinned to their sides, hardly able to move because the arm has seized up so severely. Anyone who has suffered from this condition will tell you that it isn't necessarily pain that's stopping them from moving their arm; it just won't physically go.

The reason for the arm being so stuck is that this condition causes the shoulder joint to "seize up" due to the shoulder capsule becoming tight and constricted. The shoulder capsule is a fibrous wrapper that encases your entire shoulder joint. It keeps everything in place and stops the joint from being unstable. However, in a frozen shoulder, the capsule temporarily seizes up and becomes far tighter than it is designed to be.

Although the research isn't conclusive as to whether lots of treatment can help to improve the mobility of a frozen shoulder,[6] I always think having a home exercise program to improve the mobility of the arm is a good idea. In my experience, the people who truly apply themselves to an exercise program, or get effective hands-on treatment, tend to have far better results than those who just sit and wait for the problem to go away on its own.

The self-assisted flexion exercise that follows will help you to regain range of motion if done regularly. If you can dedicate 10 minutes each day to practising these movements, that should be sufficient for you to notice some improvement in how far you can put your arms over your head, how much you can lift, and how easy it is to reach a bra strap, for example.

Be sure to check with your healthcare provider before starting any new exercise program like this one to make sure it is appropriate for you and your individual circumstances.

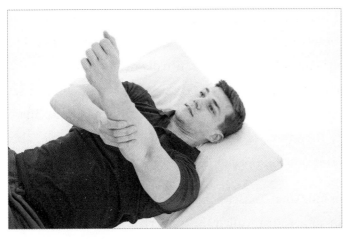

1. Lying on your bed or the floor with your knees bent, grasp the wrist of your painful arm with your good hand.

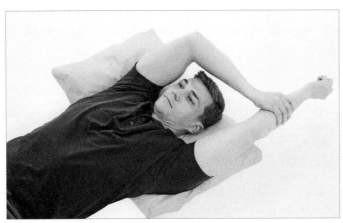

2. Using your good hand to help, take the painful arm over your head until you reach the feeling of resistance. Gently move into and out of this resistance using your good arm to help. Continue with this movement for 30 seconds four to five times a day for the best results.

The Most Important Shoulder Muscles You Never Knew You Had

If you were to conjure up the image of strong shoulder muscles, the first picture to spring to mind might be of a towering bodybuilder with boulders for shoulders. But the muscles you can see on any behemoth bodybuilder (usually the deltoids) aren't the ones that you and I should be most concerned with. There is a far more discreet set of muscles that are the origin of our impressive ability to throw, lift and climb. These muscles are also unfortunately the source of a lot of suffering for many people. This small yet vital group of muscles is called the "rotator cuff."

The rotator cuff is composed of four small muscles that sit around your shoulder blade and attach to the bone of your upper arm (called the humerus). These four muscles work as a unit and have a very important job: keeping your shoulder in its socket, as well as stabilizing your arm whenever you lift it away from your side. The rotator cuff is so called because these four muscles converge to form one large tendon that resembles a "cuff," attaching the muscles to the humerus.

When it is in good working order, your rotator cuff is a phenomenal evolutionary feature of humankind. Once upon a time, it allowed us to hunt, and being able to throw projectiles accurately gave humans the edge even over some of the most formidable predators in the prehistoric world. In the modern day, despite not needing to throw in order to hunt prey, our rotator cuffs are equally important. However, not many of us are proactive enough to look after this vital structure.

By far the most common shoulder complaints that I help my clients with are issues involving the rotator cuff. With too much stress or strain over a prolonged period, the rotator-cuff tendons can degenerate, become painful or even tear. These conditions can be debilitating. A person suffering from rotator-cuff problems is likely to struggle with lifting their arm, never mind throwing something. While this isn't as devastating as it would have been in the land of the saber-toothed tiger, it can certainly affect our quality of life in the modern world quite dramatically.

Rotator-cuff problems are often extremely painful, as anyone who's suffered from one will attest. They are a leading cause of loss of sleep, which only hampers recovery further. And what makes matters worse is that they are also stubborn to treat! So, you're far better off avoiding them in the first place if you can help it.

One fantastic way of avoiding problems with the rotator cuff is to maintain the strength of these important muscles. Strong muscles lead to strong tendons, resistant to shock and the effects of aging alike.[7] It's easy to pretend that, because you don't have shoulder pain right now, you're probably fine. But this is not necessarily so. You won't always feel the stress and strain put on the little rotator cuff. In rare cases, some people will even experience complete tears of the rotator cuff—imaginatively referred to as "massive cuff tears" in the medical profession—and not even realize.[8] The problem is, following a massive cuff tear, your shoulder function is now at serious risk.

You don't want to lose the ability to lift your arm over your head. You don't want to risk being unable to throw the ball for your dog, when he or she is staring at you excitedly. Neither do you want to risk many months of sleepless nights as a result of nagging shoulder pain. Far better to take out an insurance policy on one of the most important joints in your body, starting from today. The exercises on the following page will help you to do just that.

If you already have a rotator-cuff issue, which can often begin as a niggling shoulder pain that gets worse over time, these exercises can help rehabilitate the problem. As rotator-cuff problems are complex, it is best to be assessed and guided by a professional before giving either exercise a try. Only persist with them if it feels comfortable to do so.

You will need a resistance band and/or a dumbbell or small weight for these two lateral rotation exercises.

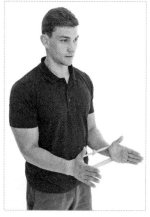 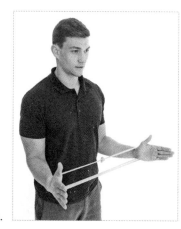

1. Using a resistance band, tie a loop and wrap the band around both wrists.

2. With your thumbs pointing up and your elbows touching your sides, pull the band apart by turning your forearms out into the band. Hold for five seconds. Repeat 10 to 15 times in a row, several times a day.

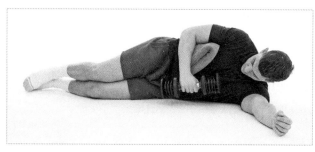

1. Lie on the opposite side of the shoulder to be worked. Tuck a rolled towel under your upper arm of the shoulder to be worked and hold a dumbbell in the hand.

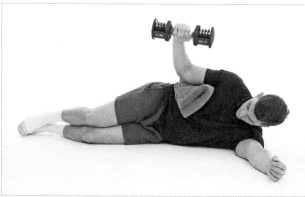

2. Keeping your elbow in contact with the towel, rotate the arm upward so as to take the dumbbell away from the midline of your body. Then slowly bring it back to the start position. Repeat 10 to 15 times, several times per day.

Getting to Grips with a Painful Shoulder

I frequently see people who have strained their shoulder after a particularly vigorous day of DIY, who then ask me what they should do to fix this. The problem is that it now hurts to lift their arm, and unfortunately almost all of the exercises you find online for shoulder pain involve raising the arm up and overhead. On top of this, it's easy to exacerbate the symptoms of a shoulder problem, leading to lingering pain for the remainder of the day.

We know exercises are very important when restoring shoulder health after an injury, but what are you supposed to do when every exercise seems to only worsen the pain? Do you just push through it? Or do you avoid them all?

Luckily, there exists an alternative that can grant relief from an irritable shoulder in the first few days after an injury, as well as starting the rehabilitation process. If you've injured the rotator cuff (*see also pages 82–84*), this simple exercise will prompt the body to start laying down new tissue and begin the healing process. And the best part is that it doesn't even involve moving your arm!

For this exercise, all you're going to do is work on your grip strength. Yes, I realize you're suffering right now with a shoulder problem, not a hand problem—but hold on a second. Recent research has shown a strong link between the muscles of the rotator cuff and the muscles we use to grip tightly.[9] Put simply, when the hand grips, the shoulder switches on.

The reason this happens is likely down to evolution. When the earliest hunter-gatherers gripped an object tightly, their next movement would often be to throw the projectile. This association has stayed with us in modern life, meaning grip and rotator-cuff function are innately connected.

So, to get the crucial muscles of the rotator cuff working without suffering the painful process of lifting your arm, all you need is to grab hold of a sponge or soft ball and start gripping.

I would recommend alternating between gripping and releasing, first very quickly (holding on for just one second before relaxing your fingers), and then gripping and squeezing for a longer period of time (holding the contraction for between five and 10 seconds). Try doing a couple of minutes of work at each tempo, then see how this affects your shoulder pain after a couple of days.

Of course, once your shoulder starts to feel better, you will need to start lifting your arm over your head again to encourage it to heal fully. If you don't eventually get the arm moving again, it will get so stiff that you'll start to lose the ability to perform this action altogether.

However, for the times when it hurts just a little too much to face lifting your arm, you'll always have your gripping exercises to fall back on to awaken the cuff and accelerate the healing process without the painful side effects of more active exercises.

In addition to your gripping exercises, here are some other things that can help to ease a painful shoulder in the early days after an injury:

- Apply heat to the painful area, which loosens tight muscles and improves mobility of the shoulder joint.

- Use pillow placement under your shoulder when lying on your back or between your shoulder and your side when lying on your side.

- If you are a side sleeper, always try to lie on your opposite side to the painful shoulder.

- Use the arm as normally as possible, unless you have been told otherwise. But if the pain becomes worse throughout the day, try cradling your arm using the other arm to take the weight off the shoulder for a few minutes.

- Asking a partner to use their fingers to press into the muscles on your shoulder blade will be painful at the time but should provide significant relief in the hours afterward for many people. See the picture below for an idea of areas to target:

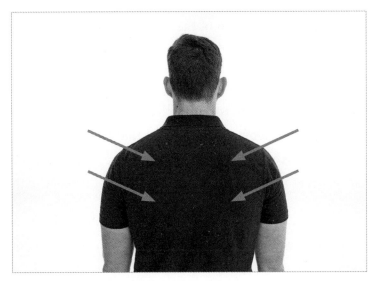

Arrows indicate the areas to press on to provide relief.

How to Release
a Trapped Nerve

Anyone who's suffered from a trapped nerve in their neck or shoulder knows just how painful it can be. The discomfort can often be felt not only in the area where the nerve is trapped but down the entire length of the nerve. This can lead to your whole arm becoming painful, not just the area where the nerve is trapped.

Symptoms of a trapped nerve can range from pain in the neck, shoulder and arm, to numbness in the hands or even a loss of strength in the affected arm. For our purposes here, we're only going to talk about trapped nerves that cause pain alone. Any trapped nerve that's giving you pins and needles, numbness or weakness should be assessed by a qualified professional as soon as possible, as it is beyond the scope of this book.

A trapped nerve can be caused by a number of different problems in the neck, shoulder or arm. No matter where the root cause of the problem is, the discomfort can be equally unpleasant.

One of the keys to releasing a trapped nerve that I often use with my clients is to gently move the affected limb in a pain-free way as often as possible. Nine times out of 10, the trapped nerve *will* eventually come free—but this process can feel like it takes a very long time to come about, especially when you're in pain! I'd always recommend an assessment from your doctor or a qualified physiotherapist if your nerve pain hasn't subsided after a few weeks.

Here are some tips you can use for relief while you wait for your body to heal and for that trapped nerve to become free at last:

Try the Following Range-of-Motion Exercises

The simple routine below can help to "free" a trapped nerve and improve mobility in the neck and arm. Only persist with the exercises that are comfortable and do not aggravate the problem.

Chin tucks

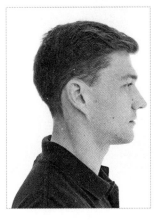 **1.** Start by sitting up tall, maintaining good posture at the neck and shoulders.

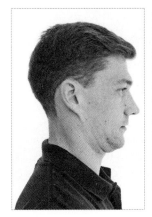 **2.** Keeping your eyes level, gently draw your chin in (so as to make a double chin), about 50 percent of the way. Hold this position for several seconds, then relax. Repeat 10 to 15 times in a row, several times per day.

Side bends

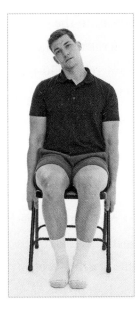 **1.** Begin by sitting up tall, maintaining good posture at the neck and shoulders. Keeping your back and shoulders steady, gently drop your right ear down toward your right shoulder, only as far as is comfortable.

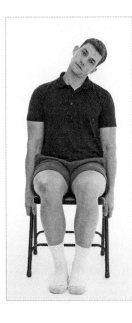 **2.** Bring the head back to the start position, then gently drop your left ear down toward your left shoulder, again only as far as is comfortable. Repeat 10 to 15 times, several times per day on each side.

Median nerve flossing

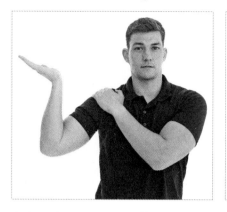 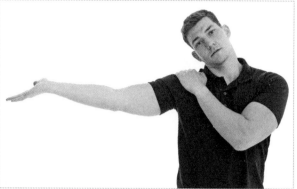

1. Start by sitting up tall, maintaining good posture at the neck and shoulders. Lift your affected arm out to the side with the palm up, as if holding a tray of drinks, and place your opposite hand on your shoulder.

2. Then, drop your ear on the same side down toward your shoulder, and as you do so, extend your arm out to the side. Bring both your head and your arm back to the start position at the same time, then repeat five to 10 times in a row, several times a day.

Use Ice on the Most Painful Areas of the Arm

Apply a cold compress, ice wrapped in a towel or a bag of frozen peas, to the painful parts of your arm or shoulder. The ice won't fix the problem, but it is nature's painkiller. It dulls the painful nerve transmissions and can bring significant relief. Go for a maximum of 15 minutes each time you use the ice and let the skin heat up to a natural temperature before reapplying. Be careful with any weak or broken skin.

Use Heat on the Neck

Ensuring you protect the skin, apply a warm compress or hot water bottle to the neck to help release any tight muscles that may be compressing a nerve. By relaxing tight neck muscles, you can encourage the stiff joints beneath to loosen up. Sometimes, this can free a trapped nerve and significantly reduce symptoms. Again, 15 minutes at a time is plenty. I recommend starting with ice on the arm (if you have arm pain) and heat on the neck.

Use Pillows

If you can feel pain from a trapped nerve when you're sitting in a chair, try placing a stack of firm pillows under the arm of the affected side. I often recommend that my patients place pillows under their arm until their elbow is in line with their armpit (with the arm slightly out to the side). This has the effect of lifting the entire shoulder girdle and relieves the pressure from the nerves around the armpit (which is where the nerves in the arm pass through to reach their final destination).

Sleep Positions

You'll want to avoid sleeping on your front as this necessitates you having to turn your head to the extreme, for extended periods; not so good for trapped nerves. If you like to sleep on your side, place pillows under your head so your head is comfortably in line with your shoulders, not dropped down to one side or propped up too high. If you prefer to sleep on your back, you might want to consider investing in a pillow that has an in-built support that sits in the crook of your neck, maintaining the natural curve of your neck as you rest. These pillows are available from most big retailers; search for an "orthopedic neck pillow" to find a good selection.

Try a Change

I've had patients with neck, shoulder and arm symptoms that I just couldn't figure out. And more times than I can count, eventually they've come back to me all smiles, saying they suddenly got better. When I enquired why, it becomes clear it had nothing to do with my treatment: "I just changed the chair I sit in every night and it went away all of a sudden!" I've heard this more than once, which is why I always recommend to my patients that they experiment with different chairs, different positions of their car seat, even a different bed, and just see how it affects their painful problem. It could well be that the simplest fix for your problem is right under your nose!

The Truth about Whiplash

If you've ever been unlucky enough to be rammed from behind while driving, you may have experienced pain afterward, typically in the neck, which we call whiplash. Whiplash is a strange syndrome—and I call it a "syndrome" because it is characterized by a set of symptoms that cannot always be easily explained.

When we are suddenly shunted forward and our neck jolts backward then flexes forward, there is the potential for damage to the delicate structures that make up the spinal column. Ligaments, tendons and even vertebrae can be damaged in a violent crash. But not everyone who develops whiplash shows signs of physical damage on a scan. It is entirely possible to have severe pain after an accident without any physical injury showing on an MRI. And, in the vast majority of cases, the people who report this are definitely not making it up.

So, how can it be possible to have such pain without any obvious evidence of an injury?

The short answer is: we don't know. It could be that the rapid flexion and extension of the neck and back has caused microscopic damage to the muscles in the neck, leading to pain and stiffness. It could be that the body has gone into a kind of "shock" reaction, locking up the affected area as a result. It could be something we have yet to discover which is causing the symptoms. The medical profession is still only just scratching the surface when it comes to whiplash.

What we do know is the following: roughly 50 percent of people who have suffered whiplash will still have neck-pain symptoms one year post-injury.[10] While it is impossible to tell who will suffer chronically the first time they are assessed, there are some simple measures that a whiplash sufferer can take to decrease the chances of ongoing symptoms. Here are the evidence-based strategies we would use at my clinic to help someone recover after a whiplash injury:

Get Anything Serious Ruled Out, Then Keep It Moving

We generally recommend a thorough assessment after any significant trauma. If this assessment rules out fractures and other nasty problems, the next best thing is usually to keep the area mobile. If left to rest, whiplash injuries tend to cause significant stiffness and tightness. Through gentle movement, it is possible to limit these unwanted effects.

Don't Be Scared to Strengthen It

The affected area will usually feel weak after whiplash. However, strength can be regained through practice and repetition. The exercises in this section of the book are often a great place to start in rebuilding lost strength.

Use Heat for Relief

Most whiplash injuries are thought to be soft-tissue related, which tend to respond well to heat. You can think of your muscles as having similar properties to plastic: when you heat them up, they become more flexible. Heat can help to reduce stiffness, tightness and pain across the neck and shoulders. Hot baths, showers and hot water bottles can all help to heat the area.

Consider Soft-Tissue Massage

Hands-on treatment from a trusted practitioner can help to free up tight areas and improve your range of motion, also reducing pain significantly.

Consider Acupuncture

I have had patients with whiplash who had pain for many years with little relief. However, even with these tricky cases, sometimes acupuncture can be the thing that turns the tide and starts to provide significant relief. The type of acupuncture I use is called "Western acupuncture" and it involves treating the area with the symptoms, as opposed to "Eastern acupuncture," which works on the basis of energy channels and chakras. Acupuncture should not be painful, if carried out correctly. It is also very safe if done by an experienced professional.

Try Not to be Afraid

There is some interesting evidence to show that people who worry their ongoing pain represents serious injury tend to take much longer in getting better. Try to dissociate the concepts of "pain" and "damage"—they are certainly not the same thing, and one can be present without the other. This is definitely true in the case of whiplash.

The Curious Case of the Stiff Shoulders

I once had a man in his eighties who came to see me in the clinic, having woken up one day with a sudden stiffness in both shoulders. He hadn't done anything significant the previous day and had no history of shoulder problems.

Looking at his shoulders, it was clear there wasn't much movement available to him. He couldn't raise his arms over his head and it hurt for him to reach out or behind himself. I initially wondered whether his stiff shoulders were caused by arthritis, but arthritis usually progresses slowly, as opposed to overnight. I treated his shoulder, gave him some range-of-motion exercises, and rebooked him for the following week.

He came back to see me the next week with no improvement; in fact, his shoulders were getting stiffer. He wasn't sleeping and he had been forced to cancel three rounds of golf booked for the past week.

I was initially confused as to why this gentleman wasn't improving—but then it dawned on me. This man was suffering with a condition called polymyalgia rheumatica. I sent him for a blood test with his doctor, which came back with raised inflammatory markers, a key indicator of this condition. The gentleman was given steroids that day, and experienced significant relief by the evening.

Polymyalgia rheumatica (or PMR for short) is a strange condition that occurs most commonly in people over the age of seventy. It is a condition that is often missed in the doctor's office, because it can appear like a frozen shoulder or a bad case of arthritis. However, it is treated very differently, so knowing about it is key.

PMR is a rheumatological condition of unknown cause, which usually affects both sides and most commonly attacks the shoulders. It causes rapid onset of stiffness and pain in the affected joints, with the capsule around the joint "seizing up" to prevent movement. There will also be a high level of inflammation in the blood with PMR, which is why a blood test is the way to detect it.

All the physiotherapy treatment in the world won't cure PMR, but a short course of steroids usually does. This is why early detection is key. The steroids can work almost instantly in many cases, with the person experiencing significant relief at the end of the first day. Of course, steroid use is a serious business and needs to be monitored by a doctor, with a plan in place for weaning the person off the medication as soon as possible.

Here are some other common symptoms of PMR to look out for:

- Extreme tiredness or a feeling of being "under the weather"
- A rapid onset of symptoms, usually over a few days
- Stiffness in the hips, often on both sides
- Feeling stiff all over, sometimes too stiff even to get out of bed
- Pain that is much worse in the morning and lasts for several hours
- Trouble sleeping because of painful shoulders
- Stiffness in the neck and problems turning the head

If you are suffering with any of these symptoms, your first stop should be your doctor. Ask for a blood test to get PMR ruled out, so you don't suffer for longer than is necessary.

Part Three

WRISTS, ELBOWS AND HANDS

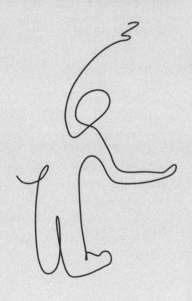

Introduction

What sets us apart from the rest of the animal kingdom, other than our superior brain power? I would argue that one of the biggest differences between us and our closest relatives in the natural world is the dexterity and effectiveness with which we are able to use our hands. Even our closest relative, the chimpanzee, lacks the dexterity of a human.

Being able to use our hands for intricate, complicated tasks is a huge asset to us as humans. But like any complex process in the body, there are things that can go wrong.

In this chapter, we will talk about how the over-fifties can stave off problems with the wrists, elbows and hands, ensuring you remain dexterous and capable as the years pass. In this section we'll look at how to ward off carpal tunnel syndrome, what tennis elbow really is, and how to ensure your hands stay strong and useful in the garden. You'll also learn how closely related the hand, wrist and elbow are, and how pain in one of these areas could indicate a problem in all three.

Use those fingers to turn the pages of this chapter and be sure to heed my advice on protecting some of your most valuable assets!

Overcoming Carpal Tunnel Syndrome

Numbness in one hand? Pain around the thumb and first two or three fingers? It could be carpal tunnel syndrome. A common overuse injury for the over-fifties, carpal tunnel syndrome is particularly prevalent in office workers and people who spend a lot of time typing or using a mouse.

As with any numbness, it's important to be checked out by a doctor as soon as possible before you try to treat the problem alone. However, if you've got a firm diagnosis of carpal tunnel syndrome, this doesn't necessarily mean you're destined for surgery, despite what you might read online.

We often see people with carpal tunnel syndrome in our clinic, and, much of the time, we can help them get back to work without them needing to go under the knife. But before I reveal how we do this for our clients, it's important to understand what causes carpal tunnel syndrome.

The "carpal tunnel" is a narrow space in the wrist between your eight carpal bones, housing a number of tendons (rope-like structures that join muscle to bone), blood vessels and nerves. One particular nerve, called the median nerve, is at risk of being compressed and irritated in the carpal tunnel by the wrist and finger tendons, which share this tight space. The median nerve's job is to provide sensation and function to your thumb and first two fingers (as well as half of your ring finger), which is why you might be suffering from numbness and pain in these parts of your hand when the nerve is irritated.

Within the carpal tunnel, there exists a battle for space between the nerve and the tendons. Through using their hands and wrist muscles in a repetitive way, some unlucky people find that the tendons in the wrist rub on the median nerve within this tight space. This can irritate, inflame and entrap the nerve, causing the classic symptoms of carpal tunnel syndrome. Luckily, there are ways we can reduce this irritation and help to "free up" the median nerve.

The best thing is, first of all, to avoid everything that aggravates the problem as much as you can. Often, it is low-level repetitive use that is the culprit—things like typing, mouse use or knitting. This doesn't necessarily mean you need to take time away from your work or hobbies; it just means changing a few things in your workspace.

The main three things to look at are your position, your equipment and your schedule.

You might want to start by experimenting with different chair heights, to adjust your sitting position. Many people undergo an "ergonomic assessment" with their occupational health department when joining a large company. However, these assessments are primarily designed to help with back and neck pain, and if your last assessment was a long time ago, circumstances may have changed. You might want to adjust your chair and see how that affects your hand and wrist. You might want to move either closer or further away from your mouse, or bring your computer closer toward you, if only temporarily. You also want to make sure your chair is the correct height. If it is too low or too high, you might be putting excess pressure on the wrist by forcing a change in angle at the wrist or elbow.

The second thing you'll want to look at is the equipment you regularly use. Do you use a standard mouse? Try a vertical mouse instead. Do you use a laptop keyboard? Try a gel pillow that supports your wrist as you type. For those of you who like to sit while you do arts and crafts, is your equipment old or outdated? Try updating it and see how that affects your symptoms. You can also use pillow placement to provide relief by raising up the wrists, which may provide enough space in the carpal tunnel to allow the tendons and nerve to coexist happily.

The third thing to address is your schedule. I don't mean you need to change your working hours; instead, look at your work pattern on a more granular scale. Break your work up into half-hour chunks. When you've finished your half an hour, take two minutes to stand up, stretch (*see below*) and rest your hands. Including regular micro-breaks can help stave off the symptoms of carpal tunnel syndrome and other repetitive strain injuries.[1]

Once you've addressed these things in your workplace or at home, you may want to look at relieving some of the tension in your wrist through a selection of gentle stretches. The tendons that irritate the median nerve belong to a set of muscles called the "wrist flexors." If you bend your wrist so as to try to touch the inside of your forearm with your fingers, you can see and feel your wrist flexors at work on the inside of your forearm.

When the wrist flexors become tight, the symptoms of carpal tunnel syndrome are more likely. So, it would make sense that stretching these muscles to lengthen them slightly can help to relieve symptoms.

Stop this wrist flexor stretch if it makes your symptoms worse and get checked by a doctor for suitability before commencing this program.

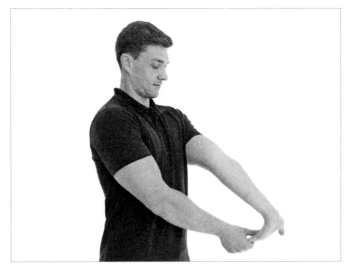

Straighten the arm to be stretched and lift it in front of you with the palm facing up. Using your other hand, pull the fingers and wrist gently back as shown until you feel a stretch in your forearm. Hold this gentle stretch for 30 seconds for four to five times per day.

The Truth about Tennis Elbow

Tennis elbow? That's just for professional tennis players, right?

Actually, tennis elbow is one of the most common conditions I am asked about in my clinic by people of all ages. And guess what? Almost all of those who ask me about it never play tennis!

Tennis elbow is characterized by a painful area around the bone on the outside of your elbow. It might be sore to touch and it is likely to feel worse whenever you use the hand to grip firmly or lift something heavy.

Now, there is something that almost always surprises my patients about tennis elbow. And that is that tennis elbow has absolutely nothing to do with the elbow joint at all. Let me explain . . .

Even though the pain you feel with tennis elbow is right on the elbow bone, the origin of the problem is somewhere else entirely. The real problem is actually in your wrist.

The muscles that control your wrist live in your forearm. They control the wrist by pulling on long tendons that run into the hand, allowing you to open jars, control a steering wheel and turn the pages of this book. These muscles live in the forearm, but some of them attach to the bones that make up your elbow via a short tendon. This tendon, rather than the bone, is the origin of the pain with tennis elbow.

Even though the problematic tendon attaches to the elbow, it actually has no control over the elbow joint at all—the tendon and the muscle attached to it control the wrist instead! Therefore, tennis elbow is categorized as an overuse injury of the wrist, not the elbow.

It is a common injury for people who do a lot of DIY; think about the action of turning a screwdriver over and over and over again. This kind of job involves a lot of wrist work, but not much effort from the elbow.

So, now we know a bit about tennis elbow, what can we do to help treat it?

With any overuse injury, there is a fundamental mismatch between the amount of work you're trying to do and the capacity of the area of the body trying to perform the work. Think about it this way: if you started training for a marathon and gradually built up from running half a mile to a full 26.2 miles over the course of two years, your muscles and tendons would likely be strong enough to cope with the demands you're asking of them. However, if you got up off the couch today and decided to run 26.2 miles right off the bat, how do you think your body would respond? It wouldn't like it, not one bit!

The same principle is often at work for people who develop tennis elbow. They go from not using their wrists very much, to suddenly using a screwdriver for four hours at a time while trying to build that new flat-pack wardrobe. Either that or they just took up tennis—and immediately began playing twice a week for two hours each time.

If this kind of thing has happened to you, you're certainly not alone (I've done it myself plenty of times, despite knowing better). You're also not necessarily going to be stuck with this painful elbow, either. Opposite, I'll show you a method I use with my clients to help them recover from tennis elbow. Called a wrist extensor lift, you can use it to strengthen your wrist muscles and recover from tennis elbow. It's a good idea to lay off the DIY for a few weeks, too. However, you can eventually get back to your DIY (or playing tennis again)—just wait until the pain has resolved first!

1. Start with your affected arm supported on a table. The forearm does not move position throughout the entire exercise. Hold a modest weight in your hand, such as a small dumbbell or a tin of beans. Begin with the weight hanging down as shown.

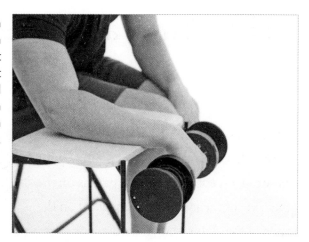

2. Use your good hand to assist your painful hand by pulling the weight upward, bringing your knuckles toward you. The forearm or elbow does not move, only the wrist.

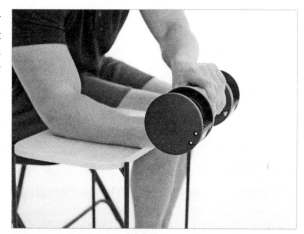

3. Let go with your good hand and very slowly control the weight back to the starting position, to the count of four or five seconds. The muscles working here are the wrist muscles that control the forearm. When you get back to the start position, repeat the exercise up to 10 times, every few hours throughout the day. If you can do more than 10 repetitions before getting a working ache in your forearm, find something heavier to hold.

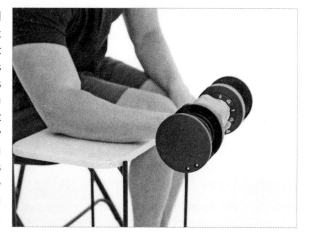

The Truth about Golfer's Elbow

Golfer's elbow is very similar to tennis elbow. This condition causes a painful point in your elbow too, except this time the pain is on the other side of the joint (the bony point on the inside of the elbow, shown here).

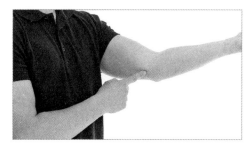

Golfer's elbow pain point

Just like tennis elbow, this problem often starts after some DIY or a long day of sport of some kind. However, I have yet to treat anyone suffering from this injury as a genuine result of golf! Golfer's elbow, just like tennis elbow, is caused by a problem with the tendons of your wrist muscles, not your elbow. If you put your hand out in front of you as if you were holding a plate of food, then try to touch the inside of your wrist with your fingers, you'll be using a group of muscles called your "wrist flexors." It is these muscles that are at the root of the problem in golfer's elbow.

Golfer's elbow is a repetitive strain injury, characterized by a problem with the tendon that joins these muscles to the bone. Because the tendon attaches the muscle to a bone in the elbow, the pain experienced in this condition is felt in your elbow, just like in tennis elbow.

One common story I hear from clients involves going to play badminton, deciding to play for half an hour longer than they normally would, then developing a very tender point on their inner elbow. This is the early stage of golfer's elbow!

Luckily, for most people, they rest the arm for a day or two and the problem disappears. However, for some unlucky people, golfer's elbow can persist far beyond a few days.

This is particularly the case for someone whose job involves lots of repetitive hand and wrist movements, giving the tendon no chance to recover.

It also unfortunately occurs for many people who decide to get into resistance training in their advancing years. The repetitive pulling motion involved in weight-training exercises can set off this kind of elbow pain and cause trouble. Despite this, I still recommend people over fifty start some kind of resistance training program (if their health allows), as the benefits are simply too great to ignore.

If you have developed golfer's elbow, fear not! There are a few steps you can put into action to reverse the problem and have that elbow feeling better soon:

- If you've just developed some elbow pain, it's a good idea to take three days' rest from the activity that caused it in the first place. For many people, this will be enough to resolve the pain.

- Right after the pain starts, it's a good idea to put ice on the painful area (be sure to protect the skin). Although there isn't usually a huge amount of inflammation present in golfer's elbow, there might be some swelling present in the first few days of the condition. Icing the area for 15 minutes at a time will help to control this, minimizing the pain and any inflammation.

- You could consider an elbow support. While this won't fix the condition, it will provide support to the joint and can limit further sprains and strains with a painful elbow if you have some unavoidable DIY to finish off.

- To fix the condition, we need to take the same approach as with tennis elbow (*see page 105*), but with a slightly different exercise in terms of your wrist positioning. We need to strengthen the muscles on the opposite side of the arm to the ones involved in tennis elbow. As the muscles involved here are different, you're going to need a different exercise. If your doctor is happy for you to try the wrist flexor lift exercise that follows, go ahead and give it a go:

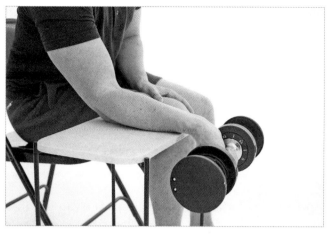

1. Start by holding a small weight in your affected hand, such as a light dumbbell or tin of beans. Rest your forearm on a table with the palm up and wrist relaxed, as shown in the picture.

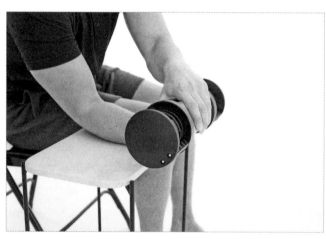

2. Using your good hand to assist the movement, bring your fingers and the weight toward you, moving only the wrist - not the elbow. Your forearm must remain in contact with the table at all times.

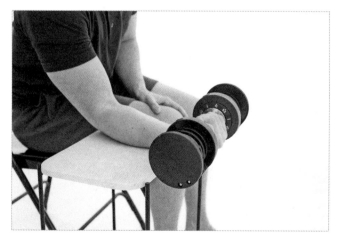

3. Then, let go with your good hand and return to the start position in a slow, controlled manner, to the count of four or five seconds. When you get to the start position, repeat up to 10 times, every few hours throughout the day. If you can do more than 10 repetitions before you get a working ache in your forearm, find something heavier to hold.

Don't Lose Your Grip!

For those reading this who are older than fifty, I've got some bad news for you: every year, if unaddressed, you're likely to lose roughly 1 percent of your muscle mass as you go through the aging process.[2] Sadly, this is just a fact of life and you're not alone; it's happening to your friends, too. The problem is, this loss of muscle mass isn't just cosmetic: it leads to a loss of crucial strength as well.[3] This loss of strength is often the driver behind many common physical problems.

Busy people like you and me use a lot of strength each day without even realizing. Climbing stairs, carrying bags and walking the dog every day all require significant use of our muscles. There are two parts of our body that we use arguably more than anything else: our hands. They are no different when it comes to the aging process, with loss of grip strength being almost synonymous with an age-related decline in health.

Our hands allow us to secure a tight grip around heavy objects, as well as perform delicate, dexterous tasks, such as doing up buttons or writing with a pen. Our hands separate us from the rest of the animal kingdom. The sheer versatility of our hands means it's our duty to take care of them.

Hands suffer with a loss of muscle mass as much as our larger muscles do. Without sufficient strength in your hands, life becomes far more difficult. There is also some alarming evidence that loss of grip strength is a reliable leading indicator of poor health and even a predictor of early death.[4] While loss of grip is unlikely to be the cause of the early mortality in these studies, it is a proxy for overall strength. Without a strong grip, it's unlikely that you will have strong arms or even strong legs. Although improving grip is unlikely to increase lifespan, it can certainly improve your health span, defined in this instance as how easily you are able to navigate the tasks of daily life.

For this reason, it is worth taking out a figurative "insurance policy" on these fantastic tools. You can do this, and thereby resist the process of aging, by strengthening your grip in some of your more idle moments. By doing so, you can be confident that your hands won't let you down in more urgent circumstances when you need them most.

There are two ways of strengthening the grip that I like to share with my clients. All you'll need for these exercises is a sponge or rolled flannel, or a soft, squeezy ball:

1. Practice the action of repetitive gripping and relaxing, squeezing your fingers hard into a sponge, as fast as you can. This helps to work the muscle to fatigue and may help to lubricate the joints in the fingers as well, protecting against arthritis.

2. Grip the sponge as hard as you can, then squeeze tightly for a duration of 10 seconds. This method helps you prepare for the walk from the shops to the car while holding bags full of shopping. This type of exercise requires the muscles to contract as hard as they can for a sustained period of time, and is called an isometric contraction.

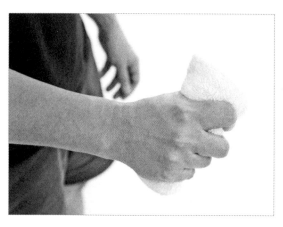

Grip the sponge and squeeze as tightly as you can for 10 seconds, then release. Repeat this movement three times.

Both sponge squeeze methods are effective and should be performed in three to four sets each day. If you have arthritis in your hands, try running a basin of warm water and plunging your hands into it while doing the exercises—it will help loosen those stiff finger joints.

Rescue Arthritic Thumbs

Pain in the thumb-side of your hand, close to the wrist? Difficulty gripping a golf club or holding a knife in the kitchen? It's possible that you could be suffering with the early signs of thumb arthritis.

Arthritis of the thumb usually appears at one of the joints in the hand that most people don't even realize exists. The picture below shows the most common joint that thumb arthritis affects:

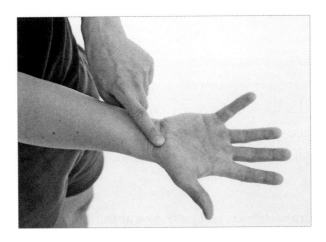

As you can see, the most common place to feel the symptoms of thumb arthritis is actually nearer to the wrist than to the tip of the thumb. We call this the first carpometacarpal joint and it is one of the most common areas of the human body to develop arthritis.

Now, many people will tell you that once you've started to develop arthritis in your thumbs, it's all downhill from here and maybe you'll soon lose the use of your grip altogether. Thankfully, for most people, the prognosis is not quite so severe and the symptoms of thumb arthritis can come and go. To be frank, it is a difficult condition to treat but, at the time of writing, conservative management is generally the best approach, especially in the early stages.

There are often plenty of things you can do to relieve some of the pain associated with thumb arthritis—and possibly limit how much further it advances. I myself have had to read up on ways of looking after my own thumbs so I can continue to practice as a physiotherapist for years to come. Coming from a professional football background, my treatment style is very "hands-on"; this certainly takes a toll on my hands and thumbs, as you can probably imagine!

If you've got arthritic thumbs, you may notice "nodules" appearing around the small joints in your thumb. They often give the joints in the thumb the appearance that they are "bigger" than they were before. These nodules appear because the body has started to lay down extra bone around the joint to spread any load that you are putting through your thumb. It's yet another way that the body is extremely clever and sophisticated in how it tries to manage stress and strain. However, these nodules can be unpleasant to look at and are a cause of great concern for many people I speak with. Unfortunately, at the time of writing there aren't any known ways for reducing them in size or stopping them from forming.

If you're suffering from stiffness and pain in your thumb or in the thumb side of the hand, here are some things that may help:

Try Using Heat

Applying a hot water bottle to the sore area in the morning and evening (being careful to protect the skin) can help to relieve tension in the hand and improve circulation in the affected area. Heat can also help to loosen up stiff joints so that you can move your hand a bit better, especially in the first 15 minutes after you wake up.

Grab a Sponge and Run a Basin Full of Warm Water

I like to give this tip to many of my clients with thumb arthritis. I often tell them to fill a basin with warm water and plunge a sponge into it. They can then exercise the affected thumb by pressing the thumb into the sponge (as if squeezing it between thumb and palm) while submerged in the water. This helps in two ways: first, you get the positive effects of the warm water, which helps to lubricate movement. Second, you get the strengthening effect of using the muscles around the thumb. This helps you to better cope with the demands of your day-to-day use of that thumb, as it should be stronger and more capable than it was before. This usually leads to less pain, too. Bear in mind that it can take up to 12 weeks before any significant strength is gained anywhere in the body, and this applies to your thumb as well.

In the Cold, Make Sure You Wear Your Gloves

When you're suffering from thumb arthritis, one of the worst things you can do is to let your hands get cold. Because our hands are an extremity, the blood from this part of our body tends to rush toward our middle whenever we get cold. This is because the body recognizes that the heart and other organs are the most important asset we have, so it sacrifices blood flow to the hands to protect our key organs. This means that, as soon as the cold weather creeps in, our hands suffer worst! By remembering to take a pair of warm gloves with you in the car or in your coat pocket, you can protect against the chills and avoid the stiffness and pain that having cold hands can bring.

Try Thumb Opposition Exercises

The thumb is a unique digit in that it is the only one that can oppose every other finger. This gives us our pincer grip. You can practice this vital movement for a few minutes every day using the following exercise:

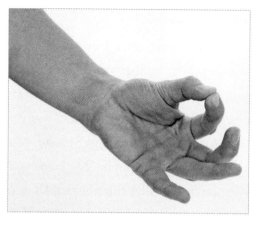

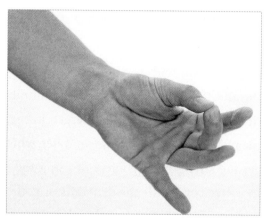

1. Press your thumb into the tip of your forefinger, holding for one second.

2. Then move through each of your fingertips in turn. Repeat this for several minutes each day.

Try Thumb Extension Exercises

The thumb is also used to open the hand wide. This movement often becomes weak in people with thumb arthritis. It can be practiced using a rubber band in the exercise below:

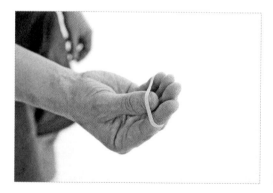

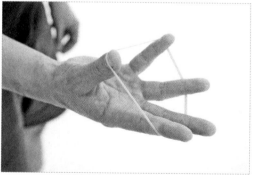

1. Placing a rubber band around your thumb and all four fingers.

2. Open your hand into the rubber band repeatedly for a few minutes. Repeat several times a day.

Preventing Repetitive Strain Injury

Repetitive strain injury (or "RSI" for short) is a plague for office and manual workers alike. RSI is a catch-all term used to describe conditions such as tendon, joint, muscle, and nerve problems that affect the elbow, wrist, and hand. RSI is common in those who use their hands repetitively, like those who spend the day typing, or who use tools like screwdrivers. RSIs can be stubborn and difficult to treat, so preventing them in the first place is worth a lot more than a cure.

In 2020, when the gyms were shut and we were all forced to find new and creative ways to exercise, I developed a habit of doing press-ups most days in the garden. That coincided with the main block of time that it took me to write the first edition of this book, so I was typing away in the day and doing press-ups at night in an attempt to remain strong.

About six weeks into this routine, I started to develop a nagging pain on the back of my wrist. It seemed to get worse after press-ups. Stupidly, I assumed it would go away on its own so I continued the exact same routine. Eventually, it got so bad I told myself I had to stop press-ups for a while. But despite stopping press-ups, the wrist problem didn't go away—it seemed to get worse after every typing session. I was finally forced to stop both activities entirely for a number of weeks and, even when I was pain-free enough to return to my writing, it took several months for the issue to resolve itself fully. This taught me a valuable lesson about preventing these issues, as opposed to trying to fix them once they have started.

The key to preventing RSI is twofold. First, you must make sure that your arms and hands are in the "optimal" position for reducing stress and strain during your working tasks. Second, you must manage the duration of time that you spend doing any one task. In my own example, some days I would get carried away on the book and write for more than four hours without stopping, even when I could feel my wrist hurting. This is a dangerous strategy and I paid the price for it! Listen to what your body is telling you.

In terms of the optimal position, we want all joints to be in their "neutral" position—typically halfway between full flexion and full extension. If you think about a press-up, the wrist is forced into full extension and held there throughout the duration of the exercise. A better alternative for me would have been to do press-ups on a closed fist once I felt the wrist pain start.

When it comes to office work, we want our elbows to be positioned at roughly 90 degrees (possibly resting on an arm rest) and our wrists to be supported on either the laptop or on a small wrist cushion (these are good for preventing wrist RSI and can be purchased cheaply online).

It is also important to keep your screen at an optimal height to avoid neck and upper-back pain. The screen you are using at work should be positioned at eye level, and should be close enough to your face so you don't have to crane your neck forward to see it.

The chair you choose should have ample lower back support, ideally shaped to match the natural curve at your spine. One thing people often miss is that, even when the ergonomic set up at your desk is perfect, you should still avoid sitting in the same position for longer than 30 minutes. In this instance, a sand timer works quite well. When the sand runs out, just stand up and stretch or go and fetch a glass of water. Even these 30 second breaks are enough to provide a postural "reset" and help prevent RSI. For bonus points, make use of a standing desk, which can be changed every 30 minutes to alternate between standing and sitting while working.

Part Four

BACK PAIN
AND
SCIATICA

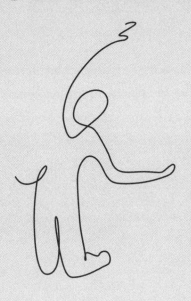

Introduction

Eighty percent of us will suffer from back pain at some point in our lives, whether it be for a day, a month or several years.[1] How we should manage back pain is still fiercely debated in modern medicine; it's the leading cause of physical disability worldwide and is responsible for an enormous number of work absences each year.

Despite the back pain epidemic, we still don't fully understand all the nuances of back pain. It may still be one of science's most challenging modern mysteries, never having been conclusively cracked or solved, despite some progress in recent years.

It is only right, seeing as I help people with back problems more than anything else, that I include a chapter about back pain (and its close relative, sciatica) in this book. My aim with this chapter is to teach you a bit about what we do know about this problem, as well as giving you some of the tools to help with it and to prevent it, should you wish to apply my lessons. I have also included a great deal about my own approach in treating my back pain patients, sharing what I have found to work better than the average approach.

Leave your expectations and current beliefs at the door: some of the following facts and methods may surprise you . . . but don't let that put you off. Read on to learn the truth about back pain, including how the body is more interconnected than you might think, as well as some simple methods that are proven to help stop back pain and sciatica in their tracks.

The Truth about Back Pain

Through millennia of pain and suffering, we have been conditioned as humans to associate *pain* with *damage*—both physically and emotionally.

As children, when we cut our hand on the shard of glass we tried to pick up to show Mum, we felt the sharp pain and saw the bleeding from our finger. When we ran too fast in the playground and fell, breaking our arm or grazing our knees, we felt the pain associated with the damage that we caused our bodies.

These experiences stick with us forever. Quite right, too! Most of the time, our experiences ring true: when we damage the body in some way, we experience pain.

Most times, the pain we experience correlates pretty well with the level of damage to the bodily tissues involved. A cut finger usually hurts like, well, a cut finger. However, there are also times when the pain we experience and the physical damage that has actually occurred to our body *fail* to match up. And when these situations occur, it runs counter to everything we've experienced in terms of pain throughout our lives.

Take back pain, for instance. For many years, we assumed that back pain was caused solely by damage to one of the many structures within the spine. Twenty years ago, if someone came to us with back pain, we would tell them that the cause of their pain was a muscle, sprained joint or damaged disc, for example. We would say that the pain would be there for as long as the tissue was injured, and when the injury heals, the pain will resolve.

We now know that this theory is fundamentally flawed. What's more, you have probably experienced this phenomenon yourself.

Over many years of medical study, and the research into pain done by scientists and clinicians, we now know it is possible, and very common in fact, for people to experience pain in the complete absence of any detectable physical injury.[2]

This means that if you've suffered from back, neck or shoulder pain at any time in your life, there's actually a good chance that there was no physical damage present in that area, despite all the painful clues suggesting otherwise.

Fascinatingly, the reverse is also true. I have had many a patient show me their MRI scan results, showing advanced wear and tear, bulging discs and even fractures, yet the patient has no pain in these areas whatsoever. The "injuries" they had suffered were seemingly undetected by the patient and were merely incidental findings on the scan (which was often performed to rule out sinister pathology).

Although relevant to any part of the body, I have included this section in the "Back Pain and Sciatica" chapter of this book because it seems that experiencing pain in the absence of true injury (and experiencing injury in the absence of pain) is one of the most common things I see related to backs in my clinic. It is a phenomenon I witness first-hand every single day.

I recently saw a patient who had been suffering with back pain for the last nine months. She finally got fed up and decided to pay out of her own pocket for an MRI scan.

She got her MRI scan results a week later. "The report says there's *nothing* wrong with my back . . . but the pain is still there! They must have read the pictures wrong. I *know* what I feel," she lamented to me directly afterward.

But the truth is, the doctors didn't read the pictures wrong at all. What my patient didn't yet understand was that although there was no physical injury to her back, it didn't mean the doctors were suggesting she wasn't telling the truth, nor that her pain was insignificant. A scan can show damaged structures, but it cannot show pain. And we know now that pain is not only related to damage; it seems that pain can also be caused by movement problems, muscle weakness, tightness or joint stiffness—none of which show up on a scan.

After an assessment, I quickly identified the problem.

When I asked my patient to bend forward and try to touch her toes, the problem was obvious. She was hardly able to move her spine at all! She was able to reach for the floor . . . but all of her available movement was coming from her hips.

With a few small tweaks to her movement, some targeted stretches and some practice at home, my patient was able to resolve her back pain within eight weeks of our first meeting.

Now, let me ask you a question: did you wake up one day with a nagging ache in your lower back? Did it progressively get worse, despite you not remembering a clear incident that could've injured your back? This is a story I also hear all the time. The truth about this kind of back pain is that usually there isn't a strain, sprain or trapped nerve causing the pain. This story is often the exact same one that my patient came to me with.

In situations like this, back pain can be caused by a combination of tightness in some areas, weakness in others, problems with movement patterns, and even changes to the way your brain is processing signals from that area of the body. As you can see from all that you've just read, it's entirely possible that your back pain is far more complex than you might have originally thought.

But don't despair! There are many positives we can take from all this. First, back pain caused by muscle tightness, weakness, and movement problems can be solved without needing to go under the surgeon's knife. As a physiotherapist, I've built a career around this fact.

We now know that opting to have surgery for back pain before trying anything else can be one of the worst things you can do. It can even make the problem worse far more often than people realize.[3] What's more, surgery can never be reversed. For this reason, we only recommend surgery as a last resort.

Second, because of the fact that back pain often isn't caused by physical damage to your back, it might be the case that getting an MRI scan could be a complete waste of your time and money.

We can't see back pain on a scan. What we will likely see are lots of age-related changes on the results of a scan, even in pain-free people, and especially for those over fifty.[4] What this means is that it's down to the best guess of your doctor as to which structure in that MRI picture is responsible for your pain. Put simply, it's impossible for us to tell accurately if it's the issue seen on the scan that is causing your pain, or something else entirely.

The other problem is that pain can move around. We don't necessarily feel pain directly in the problem area. I've had patients who came to see me about their knee pain . . . but the problem was actually their hip joint! The same is true for your back.

There are, of course, situations where an MRI scan is a good idea. These situations are usually when someone's symptoms suggest a sinister problem might be the cause of their back pain. Signs and symptoms suggesting this might be the cause include concurrent problems with the bladder and bowel, numbness or weakness in the legs, and more pain at rest than during activity. This list is certainly not exhaustive and is one reason why it's important to speak to your doctor or physiotherapist first about any new onset of back pain. Their job is to tell you whether or not a scan is appropriate for you.

I hope this section has answered more questions about back pain than it has raised. It's important to remember that 99 percent of back pain is "non-serious"; that is, it won't kill you and it should improve given the right treatment.

As always, get any new case of back pain checked out, but try not to worry too much in the early stages, even with recurrent back pain. It's likely that you haven't damaged anything. You might just need a helping hand in identifying the true cause and some advice about getting better. Hopefully, the information on the following pages can help.

Your Guide to Lower-Back Posture

When most people consider the word "posture," they think about the position of their neck and shoulders while looking at a screen. But there is another area of the body where posture is equally important: the lower back. Posture in this area of the body is much less commonly considered, yet it can have a profound impact on pain and function.

The spine has three natural curves, from top to bottom. There is an inward curve in the neck (called a lordosis), followed by an outward curve in the mid back (called a kyphosis), followed by another lordosis in the lower back. In an ideal world, these curves should be mild and gradual (*see image below right*).

The posture of the spine is determined by a number of factors, including our daily habits, the tightness or strength of certain muscles and degeneration in certain areas, such as the facet joints and discs. The truth about posture is that there is no "perfect" posture and every person is different. However, there is such a thing as a suboptimal posture and it is this sort of posture that is more likely to lead to pain and stiffness if it is allowed to manifest for long enough.

When it comes to the lower back, there are two postures that can contribute to pain and stiffness in people of any age, but not least in those over the age of fifty.

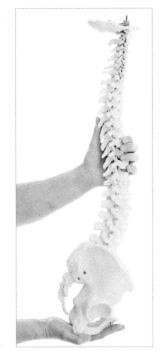

The normal curves of the spine.

1. Hyperlordosis

A hyperlordosis is an exaggerated C-shaped curve in the lumbar spine. This is also called an anterior pelvic tilt and gives the impression of a "duck bottom" in the sufferer. A hyperlordosis is a very common postural problem, particularly in modern Western societies, and it is often the result of excessive sitting.

When we sit for a long period of time, the muscles at the front of the hips become shortened and tight. One of these muscles (called the psoas major) attaches to the spine—so when it becomes tight, it tugs on its attachments and pulls the spine into a hyperlordosis.

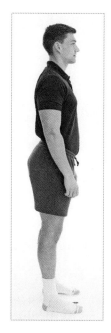

A hyperlordosis posture. Note the exaggerated curve in the lower back.

The other problem with this posture is that it is associated with weakness in the gluteal muscle group. These muscles live in the buttocks at the back of the hip and they are the opposition of the hip flexors. If the hip flexors are tight, it is very difficult for the gluteal muscles (also known as the glutes) to work as they were designed. This exacerbates the problem and leads to the hyperlordosis becoming even worse.

You might have noticed that you have the appearance of a big bottom when you stand and walk. The good news is that you might not actually have a large bottom; it could just be your posture exaggerating your backside! However, the bad news is that this posture can sometimes lead to pain if allowed to continue for long enough.

Thankfully, there is often a solution to the hyperlordotic posture. This solution involves stretching the tightened hip flexors. You can see one of my favorite hip flexor stretches on the following page.

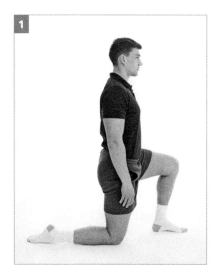
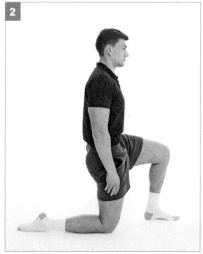

Begin by kneeling, with the knee of the leg to be stretched resting on a soft floor (1). Keeping a straight back and a tall kneeling posture, gently squeeze your buttocks and 'roll' your pelvis underneath you (2). You should feel a stretch at the front of the kneeling leg, near the hip. Hold this position for 30 seconds, repeating several times a day on each side.

The other "fix" for this problem is not allowing yourself to sit in one position for longer than an hour before getting up and moving. Just a simple stand and stretch every hour is enough to counteract the negative effects of sitting and can help to unwind tightened hip flexors.

As an anterior pelvic tilt can also be thought of as a "bad habit," it is possible to correct it over time by paying attention to it. It is possible to take note of the position of your pelvis when you walk. For many of us, when we walk our pelvises are tilted forward, causing the bottom to stick out. This can be corrected by gently squeezing the buttocks together as you walk. This should be barely noticeable to any onlooker and will have the effect of tucking the pelvis underneath you slightly, reducing the curve in your lower back. You can practice this when standing still to begin with. The following sequence shows how to do this in a standing position:

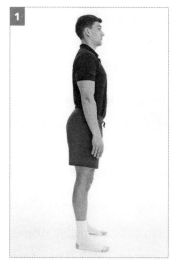
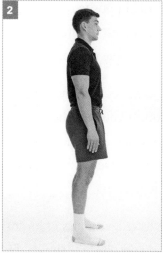

An anterior pelvic tilt causes the bottom to 'stick out' (1). This can be corrected with a subtle squeeze of the glutes when standing (2), which will also take pressure off the lower back.

2. Loss of Lordosis

An exaggerated lordosis is a bad thing—but so, too, is losing it entirely. When we lose the lordosis, we end up with a "flat-back posture" or, in the extreme, a "sway-back posture" (*see below*):

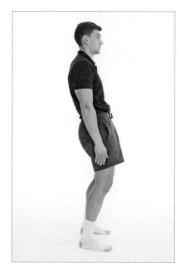

A 'sway-back posture.' Notice the loss of the curve in the lower back.

This posture is associated with the opposite of an anterior pelvic tilt, unsurprisingly called a posterior pelvic tilt. This posture is often the result of degenerative changes in the lower back and is common in people who have spinal stenosis (*see page 140*).

A flat-back posture can cause pain, because the spinal curves help to distribute load properly throughout the skeleton. If you lose these curves, the lines of force traveling through the joints become suboptimal and can cause strain over time. But fear not. If you have noticed a flat-back posture, even if as a result of degenerative change, there are often things that can be done to help it.

One thing that can be effective to relieve a loss of lordosis is to practice pelvic tilting. This can be done while sitting, and despite how simple this movement looks, it may take some practice to master. I'm demonstrating a seated pelvic tilt below:

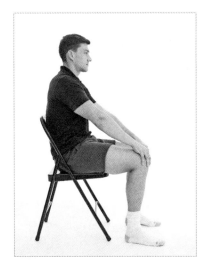 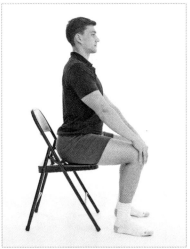

1. Start sitting in a chair with good, upright posture. Feel your sitting bones in contact with the chair. 'Roll' your pelvis forward, feeling your sitting bones move underneath you. Hold this position for a second.

2. Then do the opposite, rolling your pelvis backward and note how your sitting bones move in the opposite direction. Again, hold this position for a second. Repeat this process 10 to 15 times, several times a day.

The other thing that can help with a loss of lordosis is a hamstring stretch. Note that this exercise is NOT suitable for people suffering with sciatica as it can aggravate the problem. However, those with a simple case of postural back pain can often benefit from a seated hamstring stretch, shown below:

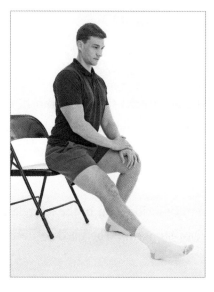

Sitting in a chair, extend the leg to be stretched out in front of you, placing the heel on the ground. Keep your foot and ankle relaxed. Put your hands on your opposite knee. Keeping a straight back, lean forward at the hips until you feel a stretch in the back of your thigh on the extended leg. Hold for 30 seconds, repeating several times a day on each side.

It usually takes months rather than days to correct a poor lower-back posture. The reason for this is that it probably took months to cause the posture in the first place! Through repeated and consistent attempts to correct postural issues we all find ourselves with from time to time, it is possible to improve our pain and stiffness—and is well worth the effort.

How Your Back Can Cause Pain in Your Leg

Have you ever heard of the term "sciatica"?

Lots of people have heard of sciatica; maybe their friend suffered from it, or they've read something about it online. But, unless they've suffered from it themselves and been forced to learn a bit more on the subject, few people actually understand what sciatica is or how it comes about.

Technically speaking, sciatica is a term used to describe pain in the leg related to the sciatic nerve. However, the word "sciatica" can sometimes be used to describe pain caused by any nerve in the leg.

The sciatic nerve is the longest, thickest nerve in the human body. It starts in the lower back, originating as nerve roots branching off from the spinal cord, and runs all the way down the back of the leg as far as the toes. You have one sciatic nerve in each leg, and it's roughly 2.5cm (1in) in diameter at its widest point.

The sciatic nerve is very important. It allows us to use our legs to walk, as well as feel sensation in our feet. But when the sciatic nerve becomes trapped, irritated or pinched, it can produce pain that runs all the way down the back of the leg, sometimes into the foot. It can also cause pins and needles or numbness in the feet and, in worse cases, weakness in some of the leg and foot muscles.

So, what causes this nerve to get trapped or irritated?

Almost always, the root cause of the problem is actually occurring in the person's lower back.

When the sciatic nerve branches off from the spinal cord to run down the leg, it must pass through some very tight spaces in the spine. If there's a problem with one of the joints or discs in your lower back, the nerve can get pinched in these tight spaces. One thing is very clear when it comes to nerves: they do not like to be touched. So, when the nerve is pressed on, trapped or irritated in the spine, this causes sciatica—and, as anyone who's suffered from this problem can attest to, it can be incredibly painful!

The structures or injuries in your back that can cause sciatica include a bulging or herniated disc (*see also page 135*), spinal stenosis (*see also page 140*), arthritis and structural changes such as a spondylolisthesis. Sciatica can also arise from "mechanical" causes, where there is no detectable injury as such, but the sciatic nerve is becoming irritated from a fault in the way a person is moving.

Another place the nerve can get trapped or irritated is in your bottom. Did you know that we put pressure on the sciatic nerve every time we sit on a chair or the toilet? You can test this out yourself by sitting on the toilet for a prolonged period of time and seeing what happens; I'll bet you end up with pins and needles in your feet when you stand up again! That's the sciatic nerve being compressed by the hard toilet seat.

Usually, we can cope with a bit of pressure on the sciatic nerve. But if we have tight bottom muscles, the sciatic nerve can get trapped here too. This is discussed in more detail in "The Elusive Piriformis Syndrome" section of this book (*see page 143*).

It's very difficult for you to self-diagnose where your sciatica is coming from. That's why it's important to be looked at by a doctor or physiotherapist who can work out where the problem originates and make a plan to treat it. However, to give you some clues as to where your sciatica might be coming from, here are some stories from the clinic:

The Bulging Disc

By far the most common cause of sciatica, an injury to the discs in the spine (shown in more detail in the next section) accounts for roughly 70 percent of cases of sciatica. And, in an ironic story, since publishing the first edition of this book, this author has suffered from this exact injury.

In February 2023, I had just returned to work from a two-week holiday where I had no access to a gym, meaning I had missed out on my usual weight-training routine for a lot longer than I would usually allow. Anxious to get back into it upon my return, on my first session back I hurriedly loaded up the bar to what I was previously lifting, ready to jump straight into deadlifts (lifting a heavy weight from the floor). Set number one felt hard, but I decided to stick with the same weight. Then, in set number two . . . BANG. I felt a sudden sharp pain in the back of my right leg, which felt like a dog biting me and not letting go. Ever the optimist, I refused to believe I had just injured my back, given that I had no back pain whatsoever. I wanted to believe that I had just tweaked my hamstring. However, that night, my entire right leg went numb—meaning the evidence was too great to ignore.

Thankfully, this story has a happy ending. Although it took four months to fully resolve the pain, I followed my own advice (although physios are notoriously bad at doing so!) and the sciatica went away. I am now back to my usual routine, without any kind of long-standing hindrance (although I am still careful with deadlifts).

The most interesting thing about this injury was that I never had back pain during the healing process, which is quite common. Many people with a bulging disc do get back pain, but not everyone. This is yet another example of how the body works in mysterious ways.

I fit the risk profile for a disc injury: the people who suffer with this problem are often active, more often male and usually between thirty and fifty years of age. I have worked with many over-fifties with disc problems too, but it is certainly not an "older person's" injury. Anyway, this injury is discussed in greater detail in the next section.

Spinal Stenosis

A gentleman once came to see me with pain in his back and both legs whenever he walked further than a few hundred yards. This problem started slowly and seemed to be getting worse. He found that leaning on his shopping cart took the pain away completely, as did walking up hills. Yet walking on the flat was becoming a nightmare, as was standing still in lines and at social gatherings. He had no pain when sitting or lying down, only when walking.

This was a classic case of spinal stenosis, which is a problem that occurs when arthritis in the spine crosses a certain threshold. The nerves live in tiny spaces within the spine, and when we suffer arthritis of the spine these spaces become even smaller still. Once this process crosses a certain point, the nerves are likely to be pinched in these tight spaces, leading to pain that usually affects the back and both legs.

Spinal stenosis is not a curable problem, but it is treatable. Read more about this condition on page 140.

Piriformis Syndrome

While the last two stories are about people who have problems with their lower backs, this final story is about a man with a similar set of symptoms but a problem somewhere else entirely.

A man in his fifties came to see me a year or two ago, complaining of sharp pain in his right buttock and a burning pain and numbness running down the back of his right leg. It was made worse by sitting, driving and running. He had no pain when he was walking or standing, and no pain when he bent forward or twisted at the spine. This gentleman had paid privately for an MRI scan of his spine, expecting to be told he had a disc injury. However, the MRI scan came back totally clear, showing a spine in very good condition and with no signs of anything touching or irritating a nerve root. When I assessed my client, I found an incredibly tender spot in his right buttock which reproduced the pain and, upon testing, his gluteal muscles were very weak on the right side.

This man was suffering with the elusive piriformis syndrome; so-called (by me) because this condition is far rarer than most people realize. In my opinion, it's over-diagnosed—I have only come across one or two patients where I could confidently say they have this condition. I will discuss more about this controversial condition in its own section (*see page 143*). For now, suffice to say that if you have been diagnosed with piriformis syndrome, I would continue to keep an open mind for something else being the true cause of your problem.

Of course, there are many more issues that can lead to sciatica, including other conditions that masquerade as sciatic nerve pain, but these are just the three that I am asked most frequently about. In the next few sections, we are going to look at these issues in more detail. I'll also share some of my most effective methods for treating them.

All You Need to Know about "Slipped Discs"

If you've ever suffered with sciatic nerve pain, there is a very high chance that the cause of it was a disc injury.

The intervertebral discs are tough, fluid-filled sacs that sit between the vertebrae in the spine. They are a vital component of a healthy spine and allow us to bend, twist and move. You can think of the spinal discs as having the structure of a jam doughnut. The fluid center of each disc (the "jam") supplies the vertebral bones with nutrients, with the tough outer casing (the "doughy" part) of each disc made of a strong yet flexible material called collagen. Without the discs, we would be permanently stiff, unable to bend or twist.

However, the discs are not without their issues. Over the course of a normal life, the discs are prone to developing tiny weaknesses in their outer layers. If these weaknesses get to a certain point, a "bulge" can develop, which is where the fluid center of the disc starts to push out toward the weak area, causing a bulging appearance in certain positions. Unfortunately, the spinal nerves are placed incredibly close to the discs and, if a disc bulge in the lower back touches a nerve, it can lead to pain in the leg called "sciatica."

If a disc bulge continues to worsen, it can develop into something called a "herniated" or "prolapsed" disc, which is sometimes colloquially known as a "slipped disc." This is when the fluid center has been squeezed out of the disc, often leaking into the area where the nerves live. This can cause an array of symptoms including sciatica, numbness, and weakness in the lower limb.

Now, this all sounds very scary. But there are some important things to know about disc injuries.

First, disc injuries are incredibly common—and many people will never know they have one. In a 2015 study, it was shown that 84 percent of people over eighty years old (who reported no back or leg pain) had disc injuries.[4] We don't know for sure why some people get pain with a disc injury while others do not, but it is likely that those without pain were lucky in that the disc bulge or prolapse never made contact with a nerve. The discs themselves are not "sensory," which means they don't have nerves inside them that communicate pain signals to the brain. Therefore, most of us can walk around with a disc injury quite happily, as long as it doesn't make contact with a nerve.

The second important thing to know about disc injuries is that they can get better. There is a lot of misinformation online regarding disc injuries, falsely claiming that the only resolution is surgery. If this was the case, I would not have a busy clinical practice, as a huge proportion of my patients are there to get better from a disc injury (and I am happy to report that we can achieve a great outcome an overwhelming majority of the time).

The third thing that anyone with a disc injury should know is that it may take a long time for the injury to heal. The discs do not have a great blood supply, meaning that healing can be slow. However, there are things that can be done to accelerate the rate at which disc injuries heal. I have made a list of ideas below which tend to work well for my patients:

Where Possible, Keep the Spine Mobile

It may hurt to bend and twist when you have a disc injury, but preventing stiffness is important. My advice to people with a disc injury is to avoid painful movements of the spine temporarily, but to do as much pain-free spinal movement as possible. My theory is that this increases the rate of blood flow to the disc and accelerates healing.

Follow the "Golden Rule" When Choosing Exercises

Exercises are important for a disc injury—but choosing the wrong exercises can set you back. The Golden Rule I tell my clients is to avoid any exercises that make your pain worse, either during the exercise or in the 12-hour period afterward. For most people, an assessment from a professional is the best way to get the right exercises, but I have shared a few of my favorite exercises in the following pages.

Keep Walking

Walking is a vital exercise for people with a disc injury. It helps to increase blood flow to the disc, decreases stiffness and helps to maintain strength. It is one of the most important evidence-based things you can do to help accelerate recovery.[5]

Avoid Hamstring Stretches

Hamstring stretches are a huge no-go for people with a disc injury, because they simultaneously stretch the sciatic nerve. When the nerve is already irritated, the last thing it needs is to be stretched. Unfortunately, I meet many people who have been told to stretch their hamstrings for relief, and this is a common reason for the injury not healing as fast as it should.

Take the Tension Off the Nerve

Similarly, we should avoid positions that put tension on the sciatic nerve. For example, lying down with your legs straight can be made less painful by putting a pillow under the knees:

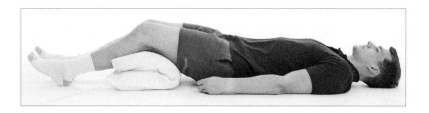

Focus on Overall Health

Eating healthily, avoiding alcohol, getting enough sleep and continuing to move as much as possible are all important factors for disc healing. As much of the pain in a disc injury is caused by inflammation around the nerve, anything we can do that will lead to a decrease in overall inflammation levels will likely be helpful.

Understand What a Recovery Looks Like

The most common symptom that occurs after a disc injury is sciatica (nerve pain in the leg). Many people also have back pain, but not all. However, during the recovery process and as the pain in the leg starts to improve, sometimes the back pain can actually get worse. We don't fully understand why this happens, but as long as the pain in the leg continues to improve, I tend to see this as a "positive" sign that things are on the right tracks. In addition, recovery from a disc injury is rarely linear and tends to be punctuated with some good days, then some very bad days. I like to look at the overall trend, as opposed to assuming we are back to square one after every "bad" day.

Get Help If You Have Any "Red Flag" Symptoms

Covered in more detail in the "When Is Back Pain an Emergency?" section on page 169, red flag symptoms include loss of bladder or bowel control, numbness in the "saddle" region, and loss of strength in the legs. These symptoms are often the sign of a severe condition called cauda equina syndrome (CES) and should be assessed by a doctor as soon as they are noticed.

Exercises

The following exercises, a cobra (*top*) and a glute stretch (*bottom*), are among my favorites for disc-injury rehabilitation. They don't work for everyone, but are often the starting point for my patients. Never persist with any disc exercises if they cause the pain to worsen.

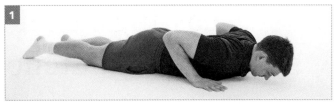

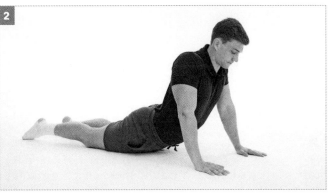

Start by lying on your front with your hands under your shoulders (1). Keeping your pelvis in contact with the ground, use your arms to lift your chest off the floor, only as far as is comfortable (2). Hold for just a couple of seconds and then return to the starting position. Repeat 10 times in a row, several times a day.

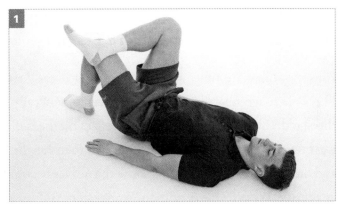

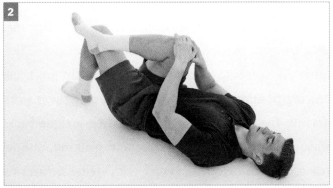

Start by lying on your back, either on your bed or on a mat on the floor. Bend both knees to a comfortable level and then cross one leg over the other (1). Cradle one knee with both hands and pull the knee up toward your opposite shoulder until you feel a stretch in the buttock (2). Hold for 30 seconds, repeating several times a day on each side.

Lasting Relief from
Spinal Stenosis

As we age, our spines age with us. The cartilage between the facet joints starts to wear away. The discs become dehydrated and lose their height. The bony surfaces of the joints become thicker, as the body tries to compensate for lost cartilage by spreading the load.

Scary as they sound, thankfully these effects are totally normal and we usually never even notice them occurring. Research consistently shows that these kinds of changes are evident in about 80 percent of the pain-free population. The natural aging process of the spine is usually not something to be feared.

However, there are times when this aging process goes much further than we would like. When age-related changes (referred to generally as "arthritis") cross a certain threshold, this can have a detrimental effect on the individual. When enough cartilage wears away and the discs lose almost all of their height, the back can become very stiff and the spaces in the spine that house the nerves become narrowed, compressing them as a result. We call this condition "spinal stenosis."

The word "stenosis" comes from a Greek word that means "narrowed." This is exactly what happens in spinal stenosis: the tight spaces in the spine are narrowed enough to cause the nerves to be compressed in certain positions. With spinal stenosis, weight-bearing positions tend to make the compression worse, simply due to the effects of gravity. The symptoms of this condition include back pain and burning in the legs, which gets worse with standing and walking, although it can usually be instantly relieved by sitting down. People with spinal stenosis tend to find their symptoms can also be relieved by leaning forward, which is why pushing a shopping cart can be a welcome activity.

The reason why sitting down and leaning forward tends to relieve symptoms of spinal stenosis is because of the way the spine is structured. When we lean back, stand or walk, the spine is in "extension," which means the bones move closer together and the spaces in the spine are somewhat closed up. When we bend forward or sit, the opposite happens: the bony surfaces move further apart and the tight spaces are widened. This gives the effect of increasing the space within which the nerves live, thus relieving compression.

If you have spinal stenosis, you can use this information to your advantage. Exercises and positions that put you into forward flexion are generally going to help the symptoms of this condition.

Many people with spinal stenosis find walking painful, but this doesn't necessarily mean walking is a bad exercise for this group of people. Using the seated lumbar flexion exercise below (and stopping to sit down now and then during a walk), and the knee rolls exercise on the next page can help those with spinal stenosis to continue to enjoy their active lives and walk further.

Start by sitting comfortably in a chair with your legs spread apart (1). Bend forward at the hips and lower back, running your hands down the front of your legs until you reach your natural limit (2). Hold for five seconds, then bring yourself back to the start position. Repeat five times, several times a day.

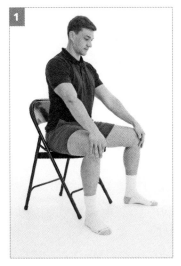
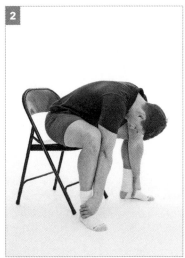

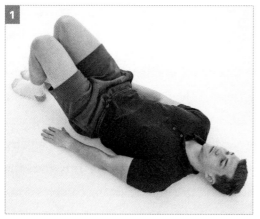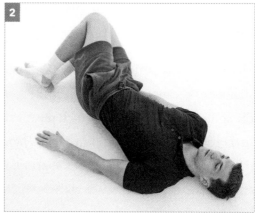

Lie on your back on your bed or a mat, with both knees bent (1). Keeping your shoulders on the floor, roll both knees over to one side until you reach your natural limit (2). Repeat in the opposite direction. Repeat 15 times in a row on each side, several times a day.

Unfortunately, there is no cure for spinal stenosis (although surgery is sometimes offered in extreme cases). However, the symptoms can be improved through proper management.

The Elusive
Piriformis Syndrome

Ironically, the cause of sciatica that I am most often asked about, but which I have almost never come across in real life, is something called piriformis syndrome.

The reason why many people think they have piriformis syndrome is because it shares many of its common symptoms with other causes of sciatica—and most people diagnose themselves in the first instance using Google, as opposed to getting an in-depth assessment from a specialist.

On the face of it, piriformis syndrome makes sense. There is a muscle that lives in the buttock called the piriformis and the sciatic nerve can pass through it. When this muscle gets tight, it pinches on the sciatic nerve, causing buttock and leg pain. The piriformis definitely exists, and in many people this area feels tight. So far, so good.

However, the chance of seeing piriformis syndrome in the wild drastically reduces once you learn that only a handful of people have the anatomy to allow its existence. I mentioned earlier that a branch of the sciatic nerve can pass through the piriformis—but this only happens in roughly 33 percent of the population.[6] For the other 67 percent, the sciatic nerve passes quite happily underneath the muscle, away from harm. This means that only a relatively small number of people even have the potential to suffer from this condition, as opposed to everyone being at risk from problems such as a disc injury.

Next, piriformis syndrome is not that common, because for it to occur, the piriformis would have to become tight for a reason. This muscle must be subjected to severe punishment or overuse for it to become tight enough to compress the sciatic nerve. While possible, it is not as easy to do this as the internet would have you believe.

Third, many people are misdiagnosed as having piriformis syndrome because there are lots of other conditions that can masquerade as this issue. Take a disc injury, for example. It is a myth that a person will always feel pain in their back when suffering with a disc injury. In many cases, someone with a disc injury only feels pain in their buttock and leg, which is exactly where someone with piriformis syndrome would expect to feel it. The point here being that the location of pain is not a great diagnostic tool when it comes to sciatica.

All of that being said, some people do get piriformis syndrome. Usually, there are a couple of contributing causes. The first is anatomical: as we mentioned earlier, you must have the anatomical variation where the sciatic nerve runs through the piriformis to be at risk. The second is mechanical, meaning there has to be a problem with your movement, which causes the piriformis to become tight and pinch on the nerve. This is where we are going to focus our attention.

The piriformis is a muscle that controls the hip. It lives in the buttock, beneath the better-known gluteal muscles (more on those later). For the hip to function properly, the muscles surrounding the joint must do the jobs they were designed for. Unfortunately, this doesn't always work out as planned.

The gluteal muscles are prone to becoming weak and underactive in many people. My theory is that this can often be a result of our Western lives, sitting in chairs and allowing poor movement habits to creep in. To cut a long story short, when the gluteal muscles become weak, something else has to pick up the slack, and that is often the piriformis. The piriformis is a small muscle, only designed to stabilize the hip, rather than be the main contributor to movement. When it is asked to pull more than its fair share, even though it can oblige for a short while, over a longer period of time this will lead to tightness in the muscle due to relentless overuse.

The symptoms of piriformis syndrome are similar to disc bulges and herniations, including buttock and leg pain, pins and needles and sometimes numbness. However, in piriformis syndrome, there are often a few key clues that help us identify the problem:

- The affected buttock will often be very tender.

- The problem almost always starts slowly.

- The person is often a runner or cyclist, or someone who does lots of repetitive actions.

- The person may find that a ring cushion relieves their pain.

- Walking usually improves the symptoms, while sitting can make them worse.

Of course, these are only clues as opposed to definitive diagnostic criteria, but they can help to indicate this condition.

Once piriformis syndrome has been identified, there is really only one way to fix it: to remedy the imbalance that caused it in the first place! If this imbalance is weakness and poor activation of the glutes, we need to build strength in this crucial group of muscles. Below is an exercise called the modified clam, which I have found to work well with people who are suffering from piriformis syndrome, when performed consistently over a long enough period of time:

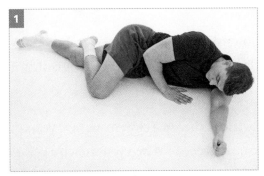 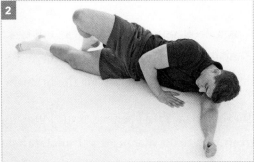

Start by lying on your side, with the affected side on top. Straighten your bottom knee and bend your top knee, hooking your ankle around the straight knee (1). Without rolling backward, lift your top knee up toward the ceiling (2). Slowly return it to the start position and repeat, 10 to 15 times in a row, several times a day.

Now, let's talk about a novel way of relieving sciatica that I've found very effective in the past for many of my clients.

My Approach to Stretching for Sciatica Relief

Through my work as a physiotherapist in my clinic, I have become known as a specialist in helping people with back problems and sciatica. One of the reasons I have had more success than most practitioners when it comes to treating sciatica is that my approach is very different to those you might find online, or in your average clinic.

Once I've assessed my patient and decided that nothing "sinister" is causing their sciatica (in some cases, this may involve getting an MRI scan done prior to treatment), I tell most people to disregard completely the typical stretches they've seen online.

Why? Because these exercises are largely ineffective for most of the people I help—and may even make the problem worse!

If you look online, the typical approach toward exercises for sciatica begins by stretching the muscles in the affected leg. The problem with this approach is that it often only serves to aggravate the problem.

The reason for this, I believe, is the following fact: it has become clear to me over years of treating patients that nerves absolutely hate to be stretched.[7] When you stretch a nerve, you aggravate the area, which can cause inflammation to increase. Unfortunately, most of the stretches recommended for sciatica don't just stretch the muscles in the leg—they stretch the sciatic nerve too.

In this way, in the process of attempting to do something good (stretching the muscles), we inadvertently do something bad (stretch the nerve). This leads either to no change, or to the symptoms getting worse. Either way, the result is not good for the person who diligently went online to search for a way to fix their problem. (This is another reason why I tell my clients not to rely solely on YouTube videos for the most part, even my own!)

Luckily, I've found a far more effective way of helping people with sciatica. It's not perfect and it isn't effective every time—but it works more than the usual approach.

Here's the approach; it's very simple. I focus my client's attention on stretching the NON-painful leg . . . while leaving the painful leg well alone.

I know this an unusual concept, but there's some recent evidence to support my theory.[8] The human body is very clever and we're starting to see proof of the fact that when you make a change on the left side of your body, in some circumstances a similar change happens on the right side, too. We aren't sure how this happens, but there may be some kind of mirroring effect going on, due to complexities in the human brain.

Another reason that could explain the positive effects of this approach is that when we're in pain, certain parts of our body compensate for the areas that aren't working well. This often means that our right side can become tight and restricted even when it's our left leg that's hurting. By stretching the right side (if the left is painful), we can often indirectly help the left leg.

This approach also means that we avoid aggravating the painful leg and everything calms down as a result.

Before I share two of the exercises I commonly use, it's important to note that these exercises aren't suitable for everyone and there's no way for me to tell if they'll help you or not. That's why it's vital you get checked out by your doctor or physiotherapist before putting these exercises into action.

That being said, let's have a look at two of the common ones I recommend to my clients with this issue:

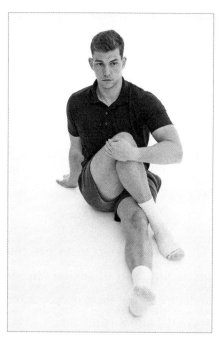

For this long-sitting glute stretch, start sitting on the floor (either unsupported as shown, or with a wall at your back for comfort). Fold the leg to be stretched (the non-painful side) over the other leg and plant the foot on the floor. Grab the knee with your opposite hand and pull toward your opposite shoulder until you feel a stretch in your buttock (on the non-painful side). Hold for 30 seconds and repeat four to five times.

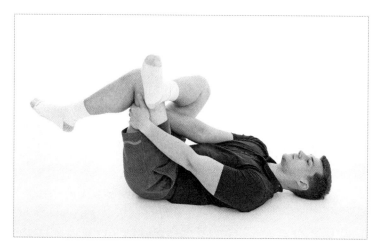

In this piriformis stretch, you are going to work your non-painful side (in this picture, that's the right leg). Lie on your back with your knees bent. Now, cross the non-painful leg over the painful leg, so the non-painful shin is in contact with your opposite thigh. Reach through the gap between your legs and pull your painful leg gently up toward you as shown in the picture. This will lift the non-painful leg into a stretch that targets the gluteal muscles and the piriformis muscle. Hold for 30 seconds, repeating five times each day.

How Sitting Affects Your Back

It's no secret that working an office job where you sit in a chair for eight hours, five days a week, 48 weeks of the year, has the potential to place you at risk of having a bad back.[9]

But why is this the case?

Surely people who keep their backs immobilized for most of the day avoid "wear and tear" or "sprains and strains" far better than more active workers?

Well, that is true to some extent. Being immobile is the only sure-fire way to avoid the kind of sprains and strains more active individuals risk suffering. However, don't let that fool you into thinking sitting is risk-free. Every job has its own unique profile of health risks. Sitting has a different, more insidious effect on our backs.[10]

For a start, in the absence of bouts of exercise done regularly before or after work, sitting for long periods of time, day after day, causes you to lose a lot of the muscle strength in your back and midriff. This area is referred to collectively as your "core."

The core acts as a sort of corset to keep your spine and midriff stable when you move. It's a vital part of your anatomy. Sitting doesn't involve much core stability, so if all we do is sit, the core gets weaker and weaker over time through disuse. This weakness can leave us vulnerable to back trouble as soon as we put any significant stress on the spine, such as when lifting something heavy from the floor.

The other reason that sitting can be bad for our backs comes down to our evolution as humans. We weren't built to sit—we were built to walk, squat and run. When we sit, several of the muscle groups in the hip and pelvis are put into a shortened position. Over time, if nothing is done to counter it, this shortened position becomes permanent.

This may contribute to the fact that, in one study, almost half of all office workers reported being uncomfortable with their work station at their job.[10]

The muscles at the front of our hips, called the "hip flexors," are significantly shortened when we sit. If we sit a lot, they remain tight even when we stand up. This can lead to a "tilt" in the pelvis, as the tight muscles pull the pelvis forward. We call this an "anterior pelvic tilt," which is a fancy term to describe the "duck-bottom" appearance that some people have when they walk around (characterized by bums and tummies sticking out).

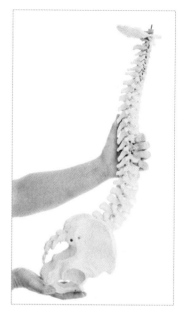

Spine model showing an anterior pelvic tilt.

This position can put stress on the back when held for a long period of time. It may be one of the most common factors contributing to back pain in office workers.[11] The problem is, this postural change happens so slowly that no one notices. However, try looking at yourself side-on in a mirror: is your bottom sticking out? Are the bony points at the front of your hips tilted forward? If you answered "yes" to either of these questions, you could be suffering with an excessive anterior pelvic tilt.

If you think you might be developing this issue, don't panic! There are a few things you can do to combat the effects of sitting and to reverse gradually the postural change you have developed.

First, it's important to try to minimize unnecessary sitting from this point onward. You might not be able to change your job, but you can minimize the length of time you spend sitting outside of work.

The other alternative is to get a standing desk for your workplace. These desks give you the option of standing up while you work. They represent a great way to break up the eight hours of sitting we may do during a working day.

If you are going to sit for long periods, it's important to stretch the tight areas at the front of the hips to prevent this tightness from building up and tugging the pelvis down or tilting it forward. There are a couple of simple stretches you can do regularly to counter the effects of sitting. One of the best ones for this issue is the hip flexor stretch, which can be found on page 126.

Control Your Core

Once only the interest of gymnasts and martial artists, the concept of "core strengthening" has sky-rocketed in popularity over the last 10 years or so, in part due to the rise of Pilates and other core-strength classes.

Pilates is a unique approach to exercise. It mainly involves attempting to use the tummy muscles (collectively referred to as "the core") to control the spine during certain movements. The goal of this exercise approach is to provide a stable base, from which you can move your limbs safely with a lowered risk of injury.[12] Although core training isn't the be-all and end-all in terms of injury prevention, having a stable core is undoubtedly important.

If your body was a building, you could think of your core as the foundations. The rest of the body (your limbs and spine) are the brickwork built on top of that foundation. If you have a weak, unstable foundation, how do you think the buildings on top of it are going to fare? Chances are, not very well.

One of the problems with modern life is that we spend a lot of time in ultra-supportive positions that feel comfortable to us. Our chairs and car seats tend to support us very well whenever we sit, which means that our tummy muscles get a free ride. This makes them lazy and weak over a period of time, which is not good. Without sufficient strength in your midriff, you cannot maintain safe control of your spine. While this might not be a problem for very basic movements, as soon as we overreach slightly, we are put at heightened risk of injury.

You might have a friend or family member who tried to bend and twist to pick up something from the floor, when suddenly they developed back pain. Many times, this is the sign of a weak core that has failed to do its job of protecting their lower back.

In this way, you can think of the core as the bodyguard of your spine. When it's nice and strong, it minimizes the harm that can come to your back when you push slightly too far in a certain direction.

So, how can we prevent the core from becoming weak? And if we are suffering with a weak core, how do we turn things around?

A good first step toward improving things would be to be more active. Walking is one great way of making the core work. This week, try to walk slightly further than you normally do by adding in one or two extra 15-minute walks over the course of the week, as long as walking is a comfortable activity for you. If you sit a lot, one great way to turn a potentially harmful position into a helpful one is to trade your chair for a gym ball. The inherent instability of a gym ball requires you to use the core to stabilize your body as you sit.

The second step to improving your core strength is to work on "switching on" your core muscles. This is a great exercise to practice in bed or on the floor, providing it isn't painful for you to perform.

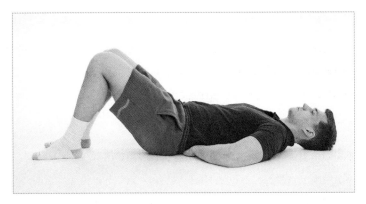

Start by lying on your back with your knees bent and your hand under the small of your back (as shown above), which should initially feel easy due to the natural curve in your spine. Now, activate your tummy muscles and squeeze your buttocks gently so as to close the gap between your lower back and the floor/bed. You should feel the pressure increase on your hand. Hold this gentle contraction for 10 seconds, then relax, repeating 10 times in a row.

Use the Static Back for Back Pain Relief

As a physiotherapist, my main goal with my clients is to improve their quality of life; this often involves working with clients to restore their mobility, improve their independence, and get them back to doing the things they love. However, one of the other very important things that people ask for when they see me is pain relief.

Back pain can be a particularly tricky issue to overcome because of its individual nature. A strategy that helps one person to experience some degree of pain relief only serves to make another feel even worse.

This is another reason why finding the right back pain exercises to do on YouTube can be a real minefield. It's always best to get exercises customized to your specific needs when it comes to back pain.

That being said, there is a position that I recommend to many of my back pain and sciatica clients that often provides some degree of relief. It's a position discovered by a leading therapist who invented an approach to treating painful problems called the Egoscue Method®.

The thing I like about this exercise is that it's very simple to do and there's little chance it will make symptoms worse. Nevertheless, no exercise is suitable for everyone, so be sure to get checked out by a doctor or physiotherapist before putting this one into action. As you'll also see, if you are unable to get down and up again from the floor, this one probably isn't for you.

This exercise is called the "static back" and it's simply a position you can get into that takes pressure off the spine. Getting into this position, even just for a few minutes each day, can be enough to ease off the symptoms of a stiff and sore back.

The goal of the time spent in this position is to allow your spine to "flatten" as much as possible as it relaxes into the floor. I usually recommend to my clients that they try to remain in this position for five minutes at a time (although many choose to stay there a lot longer—it can be an amazingly comfortable position!).

See below for the proper technique for the static back exercise:

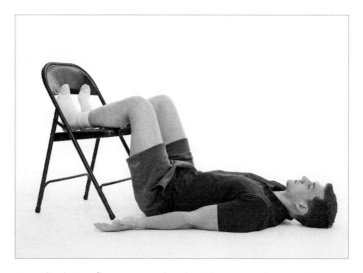

Start by lying flat on your back with your calves resting on a raised surface, like a chair. Your knees and hips should be as close to 90-degree angles as possible. Put your hands out to your sides at around a 45-degree angle with the palms facing upward. Begin to relax your spine, section by section, and feel it sinking into the floor. There should be no effort spent performing in this exercise; it is purely a relaxing position for pain relief.

How Your Feet Can Cause Back Pain

This may surprise you, but your feet could be contributing to the pain you currently suffer in your lower back.[13]

Your feet are very important. They are usually the only part of your body that makes contact with the floor. If you think about it, they support the weight of your entire body for many hours each and every day. They are like the tires of your car—without functional tires, driving your car becomes dangerous or impossible, leading to damage higher up in the axle and drive shaft.

This means that if you have a problem with your feet, there's likely to be a knock-on effect all the way up through the weight-bearing joints in the body. The main weight-bearing joints are our ankles, knees and hips, followed by the joints in our lower back. If the feet aren't doing their job properly, somewhere else is punished.

So, how can you tell if your feet aren't doing their job properly? You can get some clues by taking a good look at your feet.

- Go and stand barefoot in front of a full-length mirror and spend some time looking at your feet. What do you see?

- Do you have a nice arch in your instep? Or do your feet roll inward?

- Are your toes nice and straight? Or are some of them twisted and squashed together?

- Do you have corns, calluses or bunions?

All of these questions can help you determine how "healthy" your feet are. One of the biggest problems I see, by far, when assessing the feet of clients in my clinic is "flat feet." Flat feet is the common expression used to describe the appearance of having no instep arch. This may make the ankle look like it's rolling inward.

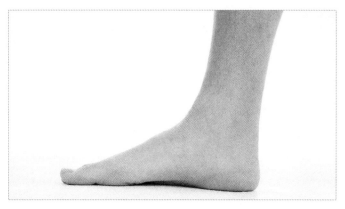

A flat foot: the instep arch has disappeared as the foot has rolled inward.

The problem with flat feet is that this condition causes a dramatic change to the way force is transmitted through the lower limbs into the floor.[14] Instead of the force of our body weight traveling straight down through the legs as it was designed, the force will now move in an angular way through the hips, ankles and knees. This places excess pressure through the joints and can lead to an increase in stress on these areas. In addition to being a potential cause of knee and hip pain, flat feet may also be a contributor to back pain in the exact same way.

So, what causes flat feet? One of the most common causes of flat feet is a loss of strength in the tiny muscles we have in our feet. Just like in our arms and hands, we have muscles in our feet, too, which help us to walk and balance. For a number of reasons, which we'll discuss later, we can lose strength in these small muscles. Flat feet can also be caused by genetic, structural problems that we inherit from our parents.

If you're suffering from flat feet, you may notice aches and pains in your hips, knees and ankles, as well as your lower back. But it's also possible that you won't feel any pain at all; some people live with flat feet quite happily their whole lives and never suffer as a result. What this means is that if you've got flat feet and back pain, it isn't necessarily the flat feet alone causing the back pain, but it could be a contributing factor.

If you think you do have flat feet, here are some things you can try to help:

Don't Always Wear Supportive Footwear

While this sounds counterintuitive, wearing supportive shoes all the time can actually cause flat feet. This happens because when we wear comfortable, supportive shoes, they do the job of the tiny muscles in our feet, meaning our foot muscles get a free ride. Because they don't need to work as hard any longer, they switch off and become lazy and weak. This can contribute to the loss of your arch, as your foot muscles aren't strong enough to maintain it any more. If you can do so without pain, try to spend at least some time walking around barefoot, especially in the house on soft surfaces like carpet.

Try an Arch Support When You're Out for a Long Walk

While I don't believe it is a good idea for everyone to wear orthotics or insoles, they can be very helpful for some people, particularly those with flat feet. If you know you're heading out for a long walk, getting an insole that supports the dropped arch can be an effective way of protecting your joints. Orthotics are little devices that you can buy off the shelf or have custom-made and put inside your shoe. They help to support weak areas of the foot and temporarily "fix" a dropped arch.

Work on Lifting Your Arch When Standing or Sitting

Try this for a few minutes each day. It's a surprisingly challenging thing to do. While sitting or standing, try to lift the inner part of your foot by using your foot muscles, without letting your toes or heel lift from the floor. You might feel as though your foot is going to cramp up when you first start practising this, but over a period of several months your feet will get stronger and be better able to support your weight without the arch "collapsing." This exercise has been shown to be effective for lifting the arch after doing it for a period of six weeks.[15]

Do Towel Scrunches to Strengthen Your Feet

There's a great exercise you can use to further fortify your feet and protect your back and lower limbs from undue stress. The best part is that it is simple to do while working at your desk or sitting in front of the TV. All you need is a towel (and a little bit of brain power to connect to the foot muscles). Take your shoes and socks off, then place the towel underneath your toes. Now, your task is to scrunch up the towel using your toes until you've pulled in the entire towel. Once you've fully pulled the towel in using just your toes, use your hands to unfurl it again and repeat three times. Don't be surprised if you get a seriously achy foot after this exercise!

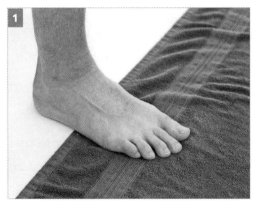 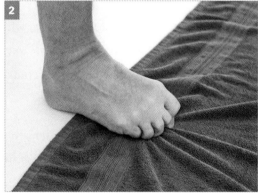

Start sitting in a chair, barefoot, with one foot on the edge of a towel that is spread out on the floor (1). Keeping your heel on the floor at all times, use the muscles in your foot and toes to scrunch up the towel and draw it in toward you (2). Repeat this movement until the towel is fully collected up by your foot, then unravel it and repeat two to three times on each foot.

The Back Pain Golden Rule

In my years of experience working as a physiotherapist, there's one principle I apply to my back pain and sciatica treatment programs that is so simple, yet I rarely hear about other practitioners sharing it with their patients. The best part is that it's an unbelievably easy way to self-guide and progress the early stages of your back pain rehabilitation program. I call it the "Back Pain Golden Rule."

If you're currently suffering with back pain, you've probably noticed that some movements or positions are especially painful. For many people, bending forward to pick something up from the floor is the most painful action they can do. For others, leaning back brings them the most discomfort. However, you'll probably also find that some movements of your spine don't cause you any pain, and may even provide some temporary relief.

My Golden Rule is simply to give my clients only those exercises that involve the comfortable movements of their spine, while avoiding any aggravating movements—until things start to improve. In this way, I help my clients to restore the mobility of their spines, reduce stiffness, and control their pain while minimizing the risk of making symptoms worse.

Anyone who has suffered for any length of time knows that it's quite easy to find an exercise that makes their pain worse, while it can be quite challenging to find an exercise that doesn't hurt and helps them to feel better. My Golden Rule improves the chances that you'll choose an exercise that is helpful rather than harmful.

So, how can you put the Golden Rule into action?

The first step is to work out exactly which movements make your pain worse. There are six "pure" movements of the lower spine, shown below. You're going to try each one in turn and see which one makes the pain feel worse.

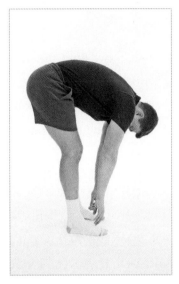

Flexion

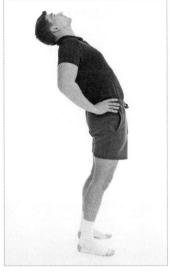

Extension

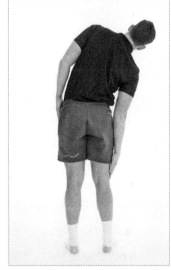

Right-side flexion

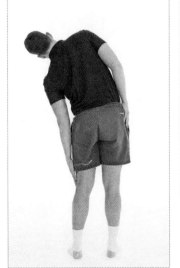

Left-side flexion

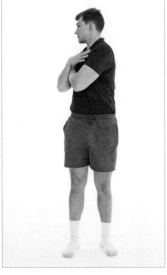

Right rotation

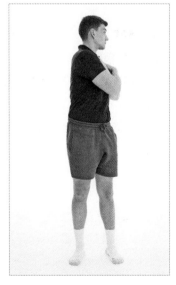

Left rotation

Let's say it's forward bending. If that's the case, you might try the opposite movement, which in this case would be gently leaning back. Try this a few times and see what happens. You might find that repeating this movement a few times actually improves your symptoms. If that is the case, you can repeat it a few times, regularly throughout the day, to limit stiffness and reduce pain. Simple, yet effective.

If you found this new movement also made your back feel worse, move onto the next movement type, which might be gently rotating the spine while sitting or standing by turning your shoulders to the left and then the right. It could be that this is your preferred movement. Your preferred movement will be different to the next person's, so the only way to know is to try them all.

Once you've chosen the movements or actions that make your pain better, just try to build them into your daily routine several times per day. I usually tell my clients to choose the most comfortable movement and repeat it between three and 10 times in a row, every two to three hours. This formula tends to work quite well. However, be sure to get your chosen exercise checked by a healthcare professional before you get started, just to make sure it's appropriate and safe for your problem first.

Once my clients' symptoms start to improve, over a number of weeks I will very slowly try to reintroduce some of the initially painful movements to their routine, in order to re-expose them to those once-problematic movement patterns and protect them from future harm. In a nutshell, along with a good deal of strengthening, stretching and hands-on therapy if appropriate, that is my general approach to treating my back pain clients.

The Most Important Muscles Supporting Your Back

When asked what the most important muscles for supporting the back are, many people would answer with the term "the core." The core, as we've already discussed, is a corset-like collection of muscles that wraps around the spine to support the entire abdomen. The core is indeed an important muscle group for supporting the lower back . . . but in my estimation, there is another muscle group that is arguably even more important for keeping your back safe and preventing pain or injury.

The group of muscles I am referring to are the gluteal muscles. The gluteal muscles make up the bulk of your buttocks and support the hip. There are three gluteal muscles in each hip: gluteus minimus, gluteus medius, and gluteus maximus. Gluteus maximus is the biggest of the three and makes up the bulk of the buttock. Gluteus minimus and gluteus medius are smaller and sit higher up relative to the maximus, just below the belt line.

The job of the gluteus maximus is to propel you forward when you walk. It acts as the driving force in big, powerful movements. Medius and minimus, on the other hand, are stabilizers, as opposed to big and powerful engines of movement. They are designed to stabilize the pelvis when you walk and provide support to the lower back during movement. These two smaller muscles have a more subtle role and appearance than the gluteus maximus, which is why they are often neglected. But forget about them at your peril, because they have a vital role that everyone should be aware of.

The problem with the gluteal muscles is that our Western lifestyles provide the total opposite of what they need to remain strong. For a start, most of us sit a lot, either at work, in the car or at home. When we sit, our glutes are placed in a lengthened position. This means that when we stand up again and start moving around, they are no longer used to being in their optimal position and thus cannot activate as well as they once could.

Sitting also causes tight hip flexors, the muscles that oppose the glutes during movements of the hip. When the hip flexors are tightened, the glutes cannot contract as well as they should. Muscles placed in a lengthened position or forced to oppose strong muscles on the other side of the joint tend to lose their "mind–muscle connection." Over time, this loss between your brain and your muscle means that even if you tried to contract the muscle consciously, it would be difficult to do so. We playfully refer to this as gluteal amnesia—because it is like the gluteal muscles have "forgotten" how to do their job.

What's more, it is easy to hide weak glutes—so much so that most people have no idea this is a problem for them, even when they develop pain. You might be thinking, "I've got strong legs, there is no way this is happening to me." But in people with "strong" legs, we often see that they are in fact "quad dominant," meaning they over-rely on their strong thigh muscles at the expense of the glutes. So it is not uncommon for me to find a gym-goer or even bodybuilder with disproportionately weak glutes, because their strong quads have been compensating. One sign that you are "quad dominant" is aching in the thighs after a leg workout—but with no such ache apparent in the buttocks.

When the glutes are weak, the lower-back muscles are able to compensate to a certain degree. The glutes stabilize the pelvis, and if they aren't doing their job properly, the strong lower-back muscles are usually happy to help—for a while, at least. However, if this pattern continues for many months (totally unbeknownst to the sufferer), the back will become tight due to the increased workload. The back muscles are primarily designed to help with big lifting movements, not endurance work. Due to them having to take over from the lazy glutes, they are doing a job they weren't designed to do. They can only go on like this for so long before a problem starts to arise.

This problem often starts as a stiff, achy lower back. You might notice a sharp pain from time to time as you bend and twist. It might cause you to worry that something might be wearing away in your back, or that you've damaged a ligament or pulled a muscle. In actual fact, it is often just the tight back muscles complaining that they are struggling to do the job that is being asked of them.

Left to its own devices, the pain might subside for a while . . . but if the underlying problem isn't fixed, it will almost always come back. This is the pattern I see in many of my clients before they come to see me. The pain comes and then disappears again, just in time to stop them from seeking help. But just as predictably, each recurring episode is slightly worse than the last. Sure, a back massage might ease it for a while, but it does nothing to fix the underlying problem (which is hiding further down in the hip). Eventually—sometimes after years—they seek help, and often kick themselves for not doing so sooner when I am able to reveal the problem to them.

I want to save you from this cycle, if I can, which is why I have included some of my favorite gluteal exercises below and on the next page. They are designed to "wake up" sleepy glutes and rebuild the mind–muscle connection so that you can use this important muscle group again. The goal for these exercises is to feel the tension develop in your hip muscles, not in your back muscles. If you have a bad case of gluteal amnesia, your back will still try to do all the work. This is why I recommend almost everyone starts with the most basic variation of these exercises, the hip abduction with resistance band (*below*), before progressing to the more difficult clam and side-lying hip abduction (*next page*).

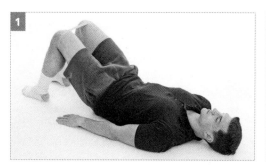
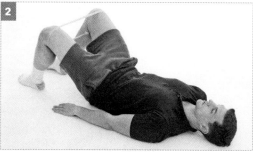

Start by lying on your back, with knees bent and a strong resistance band around the thighs (1). Squeeze your buttocks together and, as you do so, try to pull the band apart using your legs (2). How far you can move the band is not important; just pay attention to how firmly you can contract the gluteal muscles. Hold the contraction for a few moments, then relax. Repeat 10 to 15 times, several times a day.

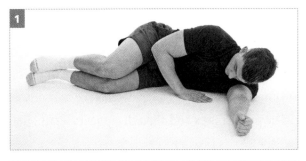

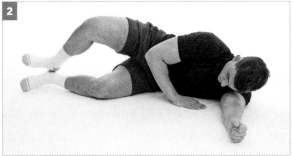

Start the clam exercise by lying on your side, with the side to be worked facing up. Bend both knees, keeping your knees and ankles together (1).
Without rolling backward, lift your top knee up toward the ceiling (2). Slowly return it to the start position and repeat, 10 to 15 times in a row, several times a day.

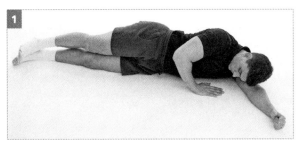

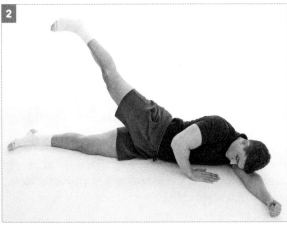

Start your side-lying hip abduction with the side to be worked on top. Straighten both knees, keeping your knees and ankles together (1).
Without rolling backward, lift your top leg up toward the ceiling and ever so slightly behind you, in a diagonal movement (2). Focus on the upper heel leading the movement. Slowly return it to the start position and repeat, 10 to 15 times in a row, several times a day.

Get Relief from Sciatica by "Flossing" the Nerve

As we mentioned previously, sciatica is the term used to describe nerve pain in the leg. Sciatica is not a "condition" in and of itself; rather, it is a symptom that can be caused by many different conditions. All cases of sciatica have one thing in common: something is irritating the sciatic nerve.

As mentioned on page 130, the sciatic nerve is the longest nerve in the body. It extends from five nerve roots that start within the spinal cord. These five nerve roots then converge into an inch-thick (2.5cm) nerve that runs through several tight spaces in the pelvis before traveling all the way down the back of the leg, under the foot to the toes.

Along its course, the nerve has the potential to be "trapped" or irritated by several structures in the back, hip, or leg. This can cause pins and needles, numbness or sciatica, but usually not in the area where the entrapment occurred. If you've sat on the toilet for too long and experienced painful pins and needles in your foot, this is a temporary experience of what it is like to compress the sciatic nerve. The compression happened between your pelvic bone and the toilet seat, but the symptoms appeared in your foot. In this way, you can get a picture of how the nervous system is connected.

Some injuries (or the process of wear and tear) can cause the already small spaces that the nerve travels through to become even tighter. This can lead to a compression of the nerve. Disc bulges, herniated discs, piriformis syndrome, and spinal stenosis are all conditions where this can occur, either temporarily or permanently.

So, that begs the question: what can be done about a sciatic nerve entrapment? Thankfully, there exists a type of exercise that can help. This type of exercise is called "nerve flossing" and it works on the premise that we are able to use certain movements to "floss" the nerve through the tight spaces in the back and legs in an attempt to free it up.

Nerve flossing (also known as neural gliding) is based on the fundamental fact that the entire nervous system is connected—so by various movements, we are able to put tension on (and take tension off) certain parts of the nervous system, thus making the long sciatic nerve "glide" within the leg or back. It's thought that this gliding motion can sometimes be enough to produce a little more space for the nerve to move within, thus reducing the entrapment and associated irritation.

The sciatic nerve-flossing technique involves alternating between two positions in a slow, careful manner. It doesn't work for everyone, but can often be incredibly effective for my sciatica clients. I like this exercise because it doesn't usually cause pain when done correctly (if it does, you should avoid it). Nor does it take a huge time commitment: 30 seconds of practice a few times a day is enough to experience positive results for many sciatica sufferers.

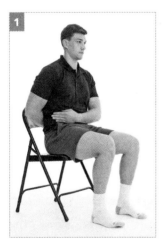 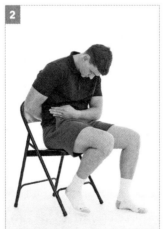 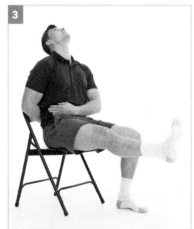

Start by sitting in a chair. Place one arm in front and one arm behind your body (1). Drop your head and shoulders down, while bending the knee of the affected leg (2). Then proceed to lift the head and shoulders while straightening the affected leg (3). Alternate between these two positions slowly for 60 seconds, several times per day.

When Is Back Pain an Emergency?

While 99 percent of cases of back pain are benign, there are some rare instances where back pain (and an associated array of symptoms) constitute an emergency. In this section, we are going to discuss some of the common warning signs to know about which might indicate that an episode of back pain is an emergency. If you recognize any of these signs, it is important to seek help immediately.

The first set of emergency signs to look out for relate to a rare condition called cauda equina syndrome (CES). This is a condition that causes a set of symptoms that indicate the lowest part of the spinal cord (called the cauda equina) is compressed by something (most commonly a disc bulge or prolapse). CES is a medical emergency and needs a review from a spinal specialist consultant within 24 hours. Here are some of the symptoms to watch out for (but note that this list is not exhaustive):

- **Loss of control of bladder and bowel:** This can entail a new onset of incontinence, inability to control the flow of urine, or a lack of sensation that one needs to "go."

- **Numbness in the saddle region:** Loss of sensation around the buttocks and genitals can mean the nerves supplying these areas are compressed.

- **Loss of sexual function:** If the genitals fail to work as they should, this can also be a sign.

- **Sciatica in both legs:** Alone, this is not enough of a symptom to diagnose CES—but it still constitutes a red flag that needs checking out.

The second set of emergency signs to watch out for may indicate an illness or medical cause for back pain. Many people who come to see me with back pain worry that they might have a tumor (or some other sinister condition) in their spine which is causing the pain. Thankfully, this is very rare. However, it is important to know what the signs are. The kind of problems we are trying to identify here are tumors, infections and cancer:

- **Weight loss:** If someone unintentionally loses 5 to 10 percent of their body weight in several months, I would be concerned.

- **Night pain:** Back pain that gets worse at night and severely disturbs sleep can sometimes indicate a medical cause of the problem.

- **Night sweats:** Anyone who is suffering from night sweats alongside back pain should be assessed by a doctor (although it is important to note night sweats can be very common in menopause).

- **Sudden and very severe back pain:** Of course, any very severe pain needs checking out by a doctor; but sudden and severe back pain can indicate an infection inside a disc or an aortic aneurysm.

- **Feeling unwell:** Generally feeling under the weather, low in energy, or having a high temperature along with back pain can all be clues that something is amiss.

- **Sudden "drop" in height:** This is a common sign of an osteoporotic fracture and can happen in people who have known osteoporosis (or individuals over the age of sixty-five who have yet to be diagnosed).

With all this being said, it is important to note that serious causes of back pain are relatively rare. This chapter is not meant to be scary . . . but it is important to know these things exist as early detection is the key to effective treatment. If this chapter saves just one person from suffering long-term consequences, it will have been worth including in the book.

Back Pain Relief
through Breathing

Breathing is one of the body's automatic functions that continues around the clock, regardless of our conscious awareness. As a simplified summary, an inhalation brings oxygen to the lungs, while an exhalation clears the body of carbon dioxide. The average person takes between 12 and 18 breaths per minute at rest, with more taken during exercise.

Breathing is an interesting action in the body because it is semi-autonomic; meaning the subconscious will take care of it when we are not paying attention, but we can override the subconscious and speed up, hold, or slow down our breath at will. It would be easy to think that the breath continues with steady inhalations and exhalations throughout the day—yet if you take some time to pay attention, you'll notice that there are occasions when you hold your breath without meaning to. This breath-holding is common at the peak of an inhalation (when the lungs are full) and has been associated with concentration. But there exists something that I like to call "inappropriate breath-holding"—and this is when we hold our breath when we move.

One of the groups of people who most commonly hold their breath as they move are back-pain sufferers. Almost all of the time, this is totally subconscious. These people tend to start their movement patterns by taking a sharp inhale, then hold their breath while they move, before exhaling completely at the end of the movement.

While this breathing pattern is unlikely to be harmful in and of itself, it has been shown to do something interesting to the central nervous system. When we hold our breath before we move, we initiate an excitatory effect on the central nervous system.[16] This has the effect of stimulating the nerves in the body, leading to an increase in muscle tone and stiffness. By holding our breath, we are telling the body it needs to be on high alert. This sounds like it might have positive implications in some contexts. Yet the problem for back-pain sufferers is that their lower-back muscles are often already on high alert. Having lower-back muscles that are always on the verge of tightening up into a painful spasm is a sad reality that many back-pain sufferers live with every day. Add breath-holding into the mix, and these people have just increased the chances of suffering one of those spasms.

The reason a back pain patient might hold their breath is due to a subconscious link that the brain has made between movement and pain. By holding the breath, the body is preparing to respond to a threat. Unfortunately, the response (the spasm) often does more damage than the threat of the movement the body was trying to protect you against.

So, what is the solution? Our goal in this instance is to try to drive down the stimulation of the central nervous system by teaching the brain that it is safe to move the body. One way we can do this is by taking conscious control over our breathing during movement. Performing breath-timing exercises, along with standard rehabilitation, has been shown to be an effective way of improving lower-back pain across a range of scientific studies.[17]

The closest thing I have found to the "perfect" breathing pattern when moving is the following: before you attempt the chosen back movement (whether that be picking something up from the floor or twisting to grab your seatbelt), take a deep inhale through your nose. Then, as you start to initiate the movement, breathe out through your mouth smoothly as you perform your chosen task. You should have empty lungs at the end of the movement. Then, breathe back in again smoothly as you return to the starting position.

I have taught this movement pattern to many of the back-pain sufferers that I treat in my clinic, especially those whose backs have a tendency to tighten up into a painful spasm. It has been a revelation to more than a handful of individuals. You can see me teach this technique on one of my videos (Video A) listed in the Resources section at the end of the book (*see page 413*).

The Tiny Muscle Responsible for a Lot of Back Trouble

There are a great many things that can go wrong with the mechanics of your spine, which can lead to pain. Tight spinal muscles, weak glutes, tight hamstrings, an insufficient core and stiff hip flexors can all contribute to mechanical back pain. But there is one tiny little muscle that is also the culprit of a lot of back pain, despite being able to consistently slip under the radar of both patient and practitioner alike. The muscle is called the tensor fascia latae (TFL) and it certainly deserves a mention in this book.

The TFL is an egg-sized muscle that lives at the front of the hip. The clue for its action is in the name: "tensor," meaning "adds tension to"; and "fascia latae," meaning the "inert tissue" that exists in the leg. Its job is to keep tension on the fascia that holds the structure of the leg together. It is also a stabilizing muscle, helping the larger muscles of the hip to produce movement. It attaches to your pelvis at one of the bony prominences on the front of the hip and onto the iliotibial band (also known as the "IT band").

The problems caused by the TFL come about when this muscle becomes tight or overused. As a stabilizing muscle, the TFL is only designed to do a certain amount of work before it becomes fatigued and grows tight over time. The TFL does the same job as the gluteal muscles at the back of the hip and also the hip flexors at the front of the hip. When we are either weak in the glutes, or overactive in the hip flexor muscle group as a whole, the TFL can tighten up, causing it to pull on its bony attachments. As it pulls down on the pelvis, it stresses the lower back and can contribute to the development of back pain.

This problem is especially common in one particular group of people: cyclists. Cycling is an activity that puts us into a flexed-hip position for extended periods of time. This alone is usually not enough to tighten up the TFL; add to the mix improper technique, though, and problems soon occur. The technique that leads to TFL tightness is the tendency to pull up on the pedals as well as to push down. When a person cycles, they should drive the pedal down with their right foot, then their left in turn. However, when cycling uphill or going for a long distance, the temptation to use a bit of pulling power with the opposite leg on the upward motion is ever present. This leads to repeated hip flexion against resistance, which is TFL's specialty. It can oblige for a while, but over time it will fatigue and tighten up. This often leads to back pain both during cycling and afterward, sometimes for a long time.

The problem with TFL tightness is that it often goes unnoticed for a very long time. This is not a muscle commonly associated with back pain, so it is often ignored in a physiotherapist's assessment. Fortunately, there is a simple way for you to test whether your TFL might be contributing to your back pain.

The position below takes the tension off the TFL. If you notice an improvement in your symptoms when you stand like this, it could mean a tight TFL.

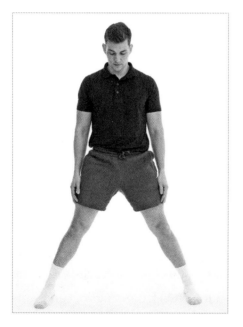

You can also try one of the movements that triggers your pain, first with a normal foot position and then with your feet wide apart. If the second attempt was less painful, that is again a positive result.

Start by standing normally, paying attention to how your back feels. Then, widen your stance so you are standing with your feet as wide apart as possible. Pay attention to how your symptoms change. If they feel easier in this new position, it is possible that your tight TFL is causing some of the problems with your back.

I experienced great results with a cyclist patient of mine once I had established her pain was being caused by the tight TFL on both sides. As a competitive cyclist, she was spending four hours a day on her bike, suffering back pain that worsened as the ride went on. I initially thought her hip flexors were the probable cause; yet when I tested them, they seemed to be fine. I tried to treat this area anyway, just in case I was wrong in my assessment. Needless to say, she didn't improve. Eventually, I tried her with the test above, which induced an instant positive result. We then changed tack and I treated her TFL on both sides with a combination of massage, acupuncture, and the exercises on the next few pages. I was also very clear in my advice on her cycling technique: she was under strict instruction not to pull up on the pedals when cycling. Within about two weeks, her two-year long bout of back pain had reduced to almost zero.

Following are two of the exercises—the TFL stretch (*below*) and the TFL release (*next page*)—I used with my patient to help her correct a tight TFL and reduce her back pain significantly.

Start kneeling, with the knee of the leg to be stretched resting on a soft floor. Keeping a straight back and a tall kneeling posture, gently squeeze your buttocks and 'roll' your pelvis underneath you (1). You should feel a stretch at the front of the kneeling leg, near the hip, on the side that is being stretched. Then put your hands behind your head and bend your trunk in the opposite direction, which will intensify the stretch (2). Hold this position for 30 seconds, repeating several times a day on each side.

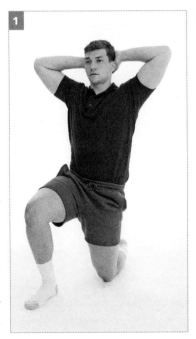
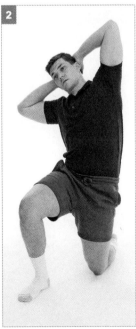

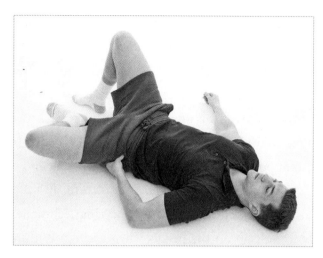

Start by lying on your back with your knees bent. Using your thumb, find the bony prominence at the front of your hip. Move 5cm (2in) below it and 2.5cm (1in) to the side. You should be on the TFL muscle. Use the thumb to press firmly on this muscle. As you do so, allow the leg to fall to the side. Maintain the pressure on the TFL muscle as you bring the leg back to the starting position and repeat 10 times, several times a day.

If you would prefer a video version of these exercises, you can find them in Video B in the Resources section (*see page 413*).

A Simple Trick for
Sciatica Calf Pain Relief

Sciatica is the bane of many a person's life who enters into my clinic. It is undoubtedly one of the most painful conditions I help people to overcome. The pain from sciatica can be present in any (or all) of the lower body, including the back, hip, leg and foot. One common area of the leg to be affected by sciatica is the calf. The reason this area is often painful is because it corresponds with two of the nerves in the spine, the L5 and S1 nerves. These two nerves are the most commonly affected nerve roots in the lumbar spine, often being irritated by disc or joint problems. When either of these nerves are irritated, calf pain can be the result.

In my time working with hundreds of people with sciatica, I have discovered a technique that can be very powerful in providing relief for people with sciatica calf pain. It is a simple mobilization that I often perform on my patients in the clinic, but there is no reason why it cannot be done as a DIY exercise.

This exercise works on the premise that the entire nervous system in the leg is connected. Just like a muscle or a joint, we can also mobilize a nerve. The nerve that supplies the outside of the calf is a branch of the sciatic nerve called the common peroneal nerve. It splits off from the sciatic nerve at around the level of the knee and then travels out toward the outer calf, before wrapping around the bone called the fibula on the outside of the lower leg.

It is my assertion that this is the nerve involved in a lot of sciatic calf pain. When it becomes irritated, it causes pain in the outside of the calf, down to the outside of the foot. Many people with this symptom come to see me at my clinic. The technique that I have found to be very useful in reducing their pain involves mobilizing the joint where the fibula meets the tibia, just below the knee. This is the area where the common peroneal nerve wraps around the bone. I cannot quite work out why this technique is so effective for many people, but my best guess is that it has something to do with the fact that we are helping the nerve in that area to glide more freely through the tight space in which it exists.

Below is the fibula mobilization exercise I use to help my clients. The movement is a gentle to and fro mobilization performed by "pushing" on the bone with the heel of your hand or thumb.

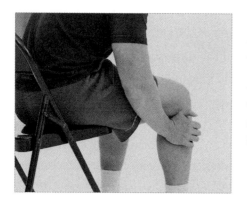

Sit on a chair. Tuck the fleshy part of the thumb side of the hand behind the little bone on the outside of your calf, just below the knee joint. Using a firm pressure, push the bone gently forward. There should only be fewer than a few millimeters (about a quarter of an inch) of movement. Relax the pressure, then repeat in a rhythmical way, for several minutes a day.

Interestingly, I recently found that the area of the leg that I teach my clients to mobilize has been used as an acupressure point for the relief of sciatica in traditional Chinese medicine (TCM). I am not educated in the Chinese medicine approach, so I cannot comment on its efficacy. However, I found this quite a coincidence and feel I may have stumbled upon something that had already been discovered thousands of years ago!

Either way, if it is going to work, this exercise tends to elicit positive results quite quickly. By repeating this exercise for a minute or two, several times per day, it is often possible to get significant relief from sciatica calf pain.

If you would prefer to see this exercise demonstrated on video, you can watch me teach it on camera in Video C in the Resources section at the end of the book (*see page 413*).

Part Five

HIPS
AND
KNEES

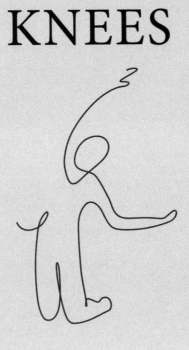

Introduction

If backs are the most common body part that I treat, knees come in as a close second. The reason I combine hips and knees together in this chapter is because of their close affinity to one another. They have a very strong relationship. For many people I treat who seek help for their knee pain, the root cause of their problem is often closer to their hips. The inverse can also be true. Knowing how closely related these two areas of the body are is the first step to understanding, treating or preventing the root cause of a painful problem in either body part.

In this chapter, we're going to dispel some myths about clicking in the hips and knees, show you how to improve your walking, and give you my single best exercise for hip and knee strength for those over fifty.

Regaining Knee Mobility

It would be easy to assume that we only lose our knee mobility after an injury that has been poorly rehabilitated. Indeed, this is one of the instances where a loss of knee mobility can be apparent. However, loss of knee mobility can also happen gradually, insidiously, without the victim even being aware of it.

Loss of knee mobility is the process of a gradual reduction in available range of motion at the knee joint. The knee moves in two directions: flexion and extension, or backward and forward. It is possible to lose range in one or both directions. A loss of knee flexion looks like someone who is unable to fully bend their knee. This might become apparent when they notice they can no longer crouch or squat. A loss of knee extension looks like someone who cannot fully straighten their knee. This is a more subtle loss of knee mobility for most people, yet just as dangerous. If you cannot extend your knee fully, your entire walking gait must change to accommodate this new restriction. I believe most people will notice stiffness in their knee if they lose roughly 20 degrees of flexion, but a stiff knee will be reported with as little as 5 degrees of extension loss.

Why do we need full knee mobility? The answer is that moving your knee through a full range of motion is necessary for many of the tasks we do every day. To walk without undue stress on other areas of the body, we must have knees that can fully extend. To climb stairs comfortably, it is necessary to have 120 degrees of flexion. Cycling without pain requires more still. Even subtle losses of mobility can be felt by the active individual.

If you have noticed that you have lost knee mobility over time, in most cases it is not too late to regain it. Through some careful practice, it is quite possible to regain those lost degrees, even if the cause of the lost range is arthritis. First, it is wise to get checked out by a healthcare professional to establish exactly what the cause is for your lost mobility; it may be an issue beyond the scope of this book. However, if you have been checked out and given the green light to start regaining your movement, simply taking your knee through the full range of motion (*as shown below*) can help.

Lie on your back, on the floor or on a bed. Bend your affected knee as far as you can, just into a sense of stiffness (1). Then straighten the knee as far as you can, pressing the knee down into the bed or floor (2). Repeat this sequence 10 to 15 times, several times a day.

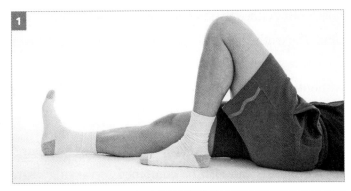
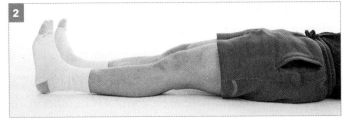

The key to making these exercises work for you is to understand that the gains are likely to be incremental. We are looking for millimeters of improvement each day, as opposed to dramatic changes. However, with persistence and consistency, it is possible to see significant changes over time. One lady came to see me at my clinic two years ago with a knee so stiff that she could only bend it to 60 degrees. For reference, that isn't even enough to climb stairs. When she sat in a chair, her leg had to be rested in front of her. Fast forward to the time of writing and she has 130 degrees of knee flexion, can climb stairs, and even ride a bike without any discomfort. To achieve these results took many sessions and a long time, but she was willing to commit to incremental improvements over time, gaining a few precious degrees each session resulting in a genuine transformation in the long term.

Regaining Hip Mobility

It isn't only a knee that can become stiff; any joint in the body can suffer stiffness over time. The truth about this process is that it often happens in a subtle, barely noticeable way. This seems to be the case for the hips, which can lose their mobility over time without our conscious awareness. Unfortunately, loss of mobility in the hip may be even more common than at the knee—and there is a good reason for that.

The hip is a ball-and-socket joint which has six "pure" movements available. These six movements can also be combined to varying degrees, making a near unlimited number of directions of movement. When taken to their maximum, each one stretches different muscles and ligaments about the joint. As we previously discussed, the only way to maintain mobility is to take our joint regularly through a full range of motion in each specific direction. Whereas we only have two directions of movement at the knee to worry about, there are a countless number at the hip, meaning it is likely that we will lose some mobility in at least one of these over time.

But all is not lost; just like with the knee, it is possible to regain lost mobility at the hip in many cases. While it would take all day to explore each and every movement at the hip, I have found a few simple movements that seem to focus on the most commonly reduced directions of movement and produce the most benefit when done regularly. Two of the most effective are shown opposite: the assisted hip flexion (*top*) and the bent-knee fall out (*bottom*). As with the knee mobility exercises, we are looking for incremental improvement, not massive jumps in mobility.

Lie on your back with knees bent (1). Bring the knee on the affected side up toward you. Grasp in front of or behind the knee with both hands and hug the knee toward your chest, only to the point of stiffness. Then relax your arms and allow the knee to drop slightly away from you (2). In a rhythmical way, repeat this sequence for two to three minutes in a row, several times a day.

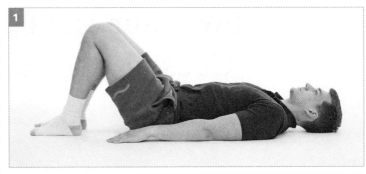

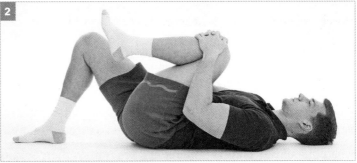

Lie on your back with knees bent (1). Allow the knee of the affected leg to drop out to the side, only as far as stiffness allows (2). Bring the knee back to the start position. Repeat 20 times, several times a day.

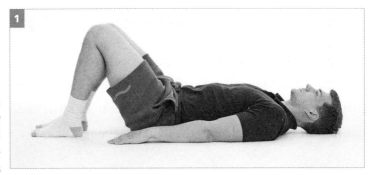

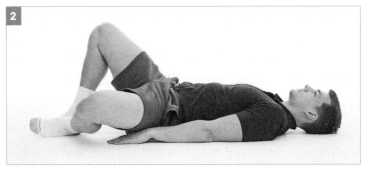

How Your Hips Can Cause Knee Pain

I've already mentioned how our hips and knees are very closely related. They are so closely related, in fact, that when there's a problem with one of these body parts, the other almost always suffers as well.

I spent a lot of time dealing with hip and knee injuries when I was working in professional football. I would see lots of knee ligament injuries, groin strains, and hamstring problems. One thing I learned as I continued to work and study was that when one of our players suffered a knee injury, there was often a problem (weakness, tightness, or stiffness) in the hip above that knee, which preceded the injury.

Sometimes, there was even a problem in the opposite hip as well.

I see the same thing in my clinic now, too, even in people who have never set foot onto a football pitch! I see people who come in with a hip problem, and when I look at the knee below, it's also stiff and sore. This means I often end up helping people with an entirely different problem to the one they thought they'd come in with!

I think it's important for me to explain how a hip problem can affect your knees, because it is something that took me a while to get my head around.

When I use the term "hip problem" in this section, I mean weakness, stiffness, or tightness around the hip joint. These are the problems that cannot be detected by an X-ray or scan but usually show up during a physical examination. It's entirely possible that you wouldn't even know that you've got a problem like this in your hip, because weakness, stiffness and tightness on their own don't always cause pain. However, after a number of months, these issues can lead to imbalances in the muscles around the hip joint. Imbalances can cause the long bone in your thigh (the femur) to fail to "align" properly when you walk, run, or climb stairs. And it is this problem that can lead to knee pain.

As half the knee joint is made up of the bottom end of the femur, when the muscles of the hip which control that bone aren't doing their job properly, it is going to affect the alignment of both the hip and the knee. That is why a problem in the hip can cause knee pain. As a concrete example, weakness in the gluteus medius muscle (*see also pages 163–166*) has been correlated with a number of lower limb conditions.[1] Once this weakness is fixed, many common knee complaints simply disappear, despite the patient receiving no obvious knee treatment.

We can also think about it in the opposite way: if there's a problem around the knee joint (the bottom part of the thigh bone), this is also going to affect the top part of the thigh bone and may lead to hip pain.

We sometimes see pain in the right knee due to a problem in the left hip, just to make matters even more confusing! Because the hips make up part of your pelvis, if one side isn't doing its job properly, the whole pelvis can drop subtly to one side. This puts an unusual pressure on both legs and may lead to pain in the opposite side.

So, what can we do to address this problem?

The first step is to diagnose the root cause of the problem and check whether it's a true knee "injury" or whether an imbalance in the hips is causing the knee pain through mechanical stress. As a side note, this is often the cause of knee pain for those who have had an X-ray or scan which identifies no obvious cause of the pain.

Discovering the true extent of imbalances in the hips and knees is difficult to do on your own. It's important to be checked out by someone who knows what they're looking for. I'd always recommend getting checked out by a physiotherapist for this, but there are also some clues you can look for at home to tell if your hip is at fault for your knee pain. For example, if you look at the way you move as you sit down and stand up from a chair, does one of your knees fall inward slightly? Ask a friend or partner to watch and check for you. If they notice one knee slightly rolling inward, that can be a sign of weakness in your hip. The same is true if you experience the knee falling inward when coming down stairs.

Once the problem has been identified, a targeted exercise program, with or without some hands-on treatment, can be the best remedy. This may mean the majority of your treatment is focused on your hips, even though your complaint is knee pain. Don't worry—once the hip imbalance improves, the knee should also get better.

Most of my clients who come to see me for this problem are relieved to hear that it often isn't arthritis or a cartilage problem causing their knee pain. In fact, for many people with this type of knee pain, if we X-rayed or scanned their knee, we wouldn't be able to see a problem at all. There doesn't always need to be physical damage for us to feel pain.[2] The type of pain felt with this problem is caused by physical stress over a sustained period of time. You can't "see" this kind of injury, but you can definitely feel it.

The key is being aware of this common phenomenon and acting early to ensure it doesn't develop into a bigger problem. Seeking early advice can prevent problems later down the line, and nip any painful stresses and strains in the bud before they get worse.

Now, we're going to talk about another extremely common yet poorly understood problem: clicking knees.

The Truth about Clicking Knees

One of the most common things by far that I get asked is: "Why do my knees click so much?"

This question is usually asked by a concerned patient who has some knee pain that they are managing quite well—but the constant orchestra coming from their knees is making them doubt their progress. Clicking, clunking and grinding noises coming from inside your knee can truly be an alarming symptom! The unpleasant natural image conjured up is that of bone grinding against bone every time you move your knee joint.

However, one thing I can assure you is that bone grinding against bone is rarely the cause of clicking knees.

First, let's quickly recap how the joints in the body work so we can understand what causes clicking in the knees. Our joints are made up of the meeting place between two or more bones. Between these bones is a wonderful substance called cartilage. Cartilage acts as a shock absorber and a lubricant, making sure the two bones don't come into close contact with each other. Another substance, which is called synovial fluid, works with the cartilage to provide lubrication between the bones and allow the joint to move freely.

Over time, the cartilage in our joints can become uneven and form tiny channels on its surface. Clicking can often occur as the synovial fluid rushes through these tiny channels, with the air bubbles within the fluid popping to give you those clicking sounds that can be so disturbing. If you've ever felt like you've got "sand" inside your knee joint, this is also the most likely explanation for that sensation.

Clicking knees is not always a benign sign and can indicate a problem, however. Sometimes, it can indicate the knee cap is failing to move as it was designed to do. When the knee cap is functioning perfectly, it slides directly up and down in the natural groove on our thigh bone. However, if we are weak in some key muscles and tight in others, the knee cap doesn't slide perfectly up and down any more because of the uneven pull caused by these muscles.[3] This causes the knee cap to "track" off to one side, and because the knee cap has left its groove, the movement isn't perfect any longer: clicking can then be heard as a result.

As I mentioned in the previous section, it isn't always the knee muscles that are at fault. This problem is yet another issue that can be caused by weakness in your hips. If your hip muscles aren't strong enough to keep your thigh bone in line, your knee falls inward and the forces exerted on the knee cap are no longer ideal. This can lead to knee-cap pain and clicking, even though the real underlying issue is up in the hip.[4]

It's very rare for clicking knees to be caused by bone rubbing against bone. Usually, bone rubbing against bone would be so painful that you'd be unable to walk, let alone put enough pressure through your legs to set off the clicking in your knees. This means I am usually able to put my clients' minds at ease when they come to me worrying that their knee has deteriorated enough to necessitate urgent surgery.

However, as with all other problems mentioned in this book, it's best to get checked out by a professional if you're worried. Hopefully, your mind will be put at ease, too.

Clicking knees aren't necessarily a reliable sign of arthritis, either. I used to treat girls as young as 16 years of age who came to my clinic with the noisiest knees you've ever heard. The noise wasn't because their cartilage had deteriorated; it was simply because their knee cap wasn't quite moving correctly. Luckily, this is a problem that we are very good at fixing for people.

One important caveat to mention is that, although clicking doesn't mean your knees are degenerating, if these imbalances are left for an extended period of time there is a possibility that your long-term knee health could suffer.[5] Knee clicking often means there is an issue with movement at that joint and, when a joint isn't moving properly, it leaves the cartilage vulnerable to wear and tear over a long period of time.

You can think of clicking knees as an early warning sign that your movement isn't quite right. The good news is that, more often than not, these problems can be fixed when caught early! The key is early detection and swift action: if you've got noisy knees, get them checked to safeguard against problems in the future.

To stop noisy knees and relieve any pain at the front of the knee, read on to the next section for some tips and exercises.

Knee-Cap Pain— What's Behind It?

Pain at the front of the knee is an incredibly common problem for many people, young and old. I'd go as far as saying that in the young people I see in my clinic, it is possibly the most common problem I help them with.

However, knee-cap pain doesn't just affect young people. This problem equally affects over-fifties too. Even though arthritis can sometimes be involved with knee-cap pain in over-fifties, the same problem that causes the pain in a sixteen-year-old can be the culprit in a sixty-year-old too.

As we previously mentioned, knee cap (or patella) pain usually occurs due to a problem with the way that your knee cap is moving.[6] Your patella was built to sit in a "groove" on top of the long leg bone in your thigh (called your femur). As you bend and straighten your knee, your patella slides up and down on top of this bone—acting like a pulley system—allowing your knee muscles to pull on your shin bone and create movement.

The patella has certain muscles that attach onto it and pull it in different directions. When everything is balanced, the patella is pulled directly up and down inside the groove and you have healthy knee movement. However, when some of these muscles pull either too hard or not hard enough, the patella may start to slide up and down outside of the center of the groove. When this happens, pain at the front of the knee can be the result.

There is a little pocket of fat called a "fat pad," which sits underneath the patella. This fat pad acts as a cushion and lubricates movement. It also has nerves within it, so when the fat pad gets irritated (by the knee cap not moving correctly), it can become very inflamed and painful.

Patella pain is often felt behind the knee cap and it can feel as if you need to get in behind the patella and add some WD-40 at times! Adding WD-40 to your joints isn't practical, unfortunately; but there are some things you can do instead.

In some cases, patella pain is due to arthritis, but try not to worry just yet. Arthritis symptoms can often be greatly improved through conservative measures, without needing to opt for surgery, injections or painkillers.

Here are some top tips for easing knee-cap pain at home:

Try Using Ice Over the Patella When It's Painful

You can apply a cold compress or ice pack to a painful knee cap to relieve some of the pain. Ice is nature's painkiller and it is very effective for knee-cap pain as the problem tends to sit close to the surface. This approach can help to calm an irritated fat pad underneath the knee cap. Be sure to protect the skin and treat your knee with ice for no longer than 15 minutes at a time.

Try to Move in a Straight Line

When we get up from a sitting position, often we're in a rush to do something, so we twist as we're rising from the chair. Try not to do this if you've got patella pain. When you twist while getting up from a chair, you can accidentally aggravate the sensitive area around your patella by causing it to move outside of its groove.

If Walking Is Painful, Try Walking in the Swimming Pool for Exercise

When we're walking on land, we take 100 percent of our body weight through our legs. In the absence of a painful problem, this is fine. However, when you're suffering with knee pain, your body weight suddenly feels much heavier. If taking your weight through your knees is giving you discomfort but you still want to get some all-important exercise in, try walking for 30 minutes in the swimming pool instead. When submerged in the water, 50 percent of your body weight is offloaded onto the water so you only need to carry the other 50 percent through your joints. This should result in instant relief compared to walking on land. The good thing about walking in the water is that it's fantastic exercise, as you're constantly pushing forward against water resistance. This means you're able to build strength (very important) without worsening your pain in doing so.

Try to Lose Some Weight

If you're a little on the heavy side at the moment, losing weight should significantly improve your symptoms.[7] I understand it can be very difficult to lose weight when you're in pain because of how hard this makes it to exercise. However, just a small change in your body weight can be noticed as a dramatic improvement in symptoms. As a general guide, I usually start to see noticeable improvements in my clients' knee-pain symptoms following around 2kg (4.4lbs) of weight loss. You can find more information about losing weight with a painful problem later in the book (*see page 308*).

Try These Exercises to Improve Your Patellofemoral Movement

Patellofemoral movement describes the relationship between the patella and the groove that it sits within. As discussed, in people with a problem in this area, the patella is not moving well within the groove, often due to imbalanced pulling forces from muscles surrounding the patella. We can improve those pulling forces with the straight leg raise (*opposite top*) and inner-range quads (*opposite bottom*) exercises. The clam exercise (*see page 166, top*) is also a fantastic exercise for this condition.

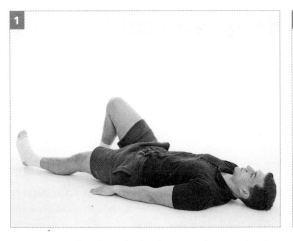 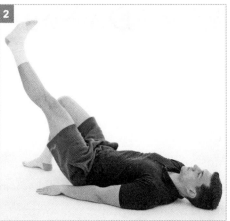

Lie on your back with the knee to be worked straight and the other knee bent. Keep your lower back flat (1). Keeping your working leg straight, lift the leg up in the air, until both thighs are in line (2). Then slowly lower the leg to the ground. Repeat 10 to 15 times, several times a day.

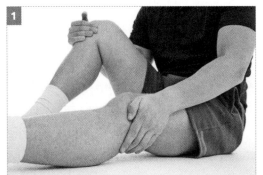 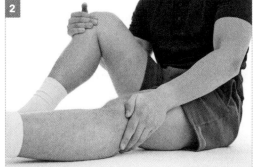

Sitting with the knee to be worked straight and the other knee bent, use your knee muscles to push down and lift your heel, feeling the muscles activating at the front of your thigh. You will notice that your knee cap slides up and down as you contract and relax the muscles to repeat this movement (1). To make this exercise more effective, you can use your hand to guide the knee cap toward the midline of the body as it moves (2).

Do Your Hips Swivel?

One of the hobbies most commonly enjoyed by my clients is golf.

Most people know you need to be able to twist from your lower back to be able to hit the ball straight and far. But did you also know that being able to rotate at your hips is also crucial for a proper golf swing?[8]

Without being able to rotate your hips, it would be impossible to get a proper follow-through with any golf swing. Your trailing leg wouldn't be able to turn to allow your body to follow the ball as you swing through.

And it isn't just your golf game that would be affected without the capacity for proper hip rotation. Swimming, walking and bowls would be very difficult without good hip mobility. At the extreme, without the ability to rotate at your hips, you will start to find even putting your socks on and getting into a car challenging.

I meet some clients who suffer groin pain when they get up after sitting for a long time in the car or at home. On closer inspection, they've lost a great deal of their capacity for hip rotation. This loss of movement can cause aches and pains when they start moving again after being at rest. If this sounds like you, it's important to act before your hips get any stiffer.

Most people have some degree of arthritis in their hips by the time they reach their fiftieth birthday.[9] Arthritis usually leads to a loss of hip rotation, long before the first signs of pain. This means you could be affected by this loss of hip movement without even knowing it!

However, no need to worry just yet. With a little time and practice, it's possible to regain some of the rotation around your hips and get the swivel back in your step.

There are two types of rotation at your hip joint. If you sit in a chair and turn your thigh bone so that the outside of your shin comes up toward you, while your foot comes off the floor (as if you're trying to touch the outside of your heel), that is the first type of hip rotation, called internal rotation (*see right*).

If you do the opposite movement, sitting in a chair and turning your thigh so that you are bringing the inside of your shin up toward you and your foot off the floor (as if you were putting your socks on), you're performing the second type of hip rotation, called external rotation (*see below right*).

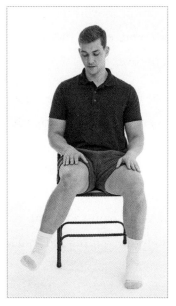

Internal rotation of the hip

We used to believe there was a predictable pattern of movement deterioration with arthritis. Early researchers believed people would almost always lose internal rotation first. However, more recent research shows this is not necessarily the case.[10]

While you may find you struggle with at least one of these movements, it is possible to notice at least some improvements in the range of motion at the hip joint simply by practising these actions from a sitting position, consistently, over a long period of time. It does take time and you may progress so slowly that you hardly notice, but most of my clients who

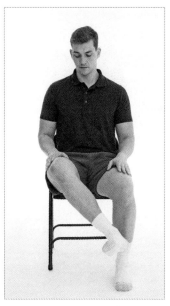

External rotation of the hip

commit to working on these movements do realize, over time, that getting into a car becomes easier, they have less trouble with socks and, sometimes, their golf game even improves too!

The following supine rotation of the hip exercise should be done very carefully to avoid aggravating already painful hips, but it's worth speaking to a doctor or physiotherapist before putting this one into action. For hips that are painful, just move within a comfortable range. If you have hips that aren't painful but are very stiff, you could try gently pushing into these stiff ranges and slowly building up. Stop at any point if you develop pain in the hip or groin, but if it's comfortable, this should help you regain some of your hip movement.

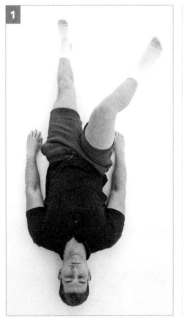
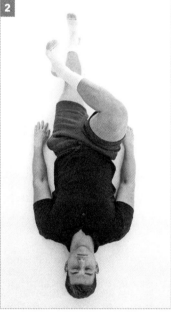

Lie on your back on the bed or the floor. Bring one knee up so your foot is off the floor. Then, keeping your knee at 90 degrees, rotate your leg first internally (1), then externally (2). Repeat 10 times slowly in each direction, for three sets on each leg.

Trouble with Walking?
Look to Your Pelvis

For you to be able to walk well, there must be synergy between your feet, ankles, knees and hips. These joints all move in concert to propel us forward as we walk. When we take a step, we begin by generating tension in our foot as it strikes the ground. Strong hip muscles then work to drive our leg behind us, as our knee muscles work to extend our knee. Finally, our calf muscles propel us forward as we push off through our toes.

None of these movements would be possible if we didn't have a solid, stable foundation from which to produce them. We've already spoken about the core being the muscular foundation of the body, but there is a bony foundation, too: your pelvis.

The pelvis sits in the middle of the human body and provides an attachment point for 36 different muscles. The pulling forces these muscles exert on the pelvis make up something called pelvic control. Pelvic control describes the position of the pelvis as we walk and move. There is an optimal position for the pelvis to be in at any given time. If your pelvis is in this position for most of the time due to equal and proportional forces acting upon it, we call this good pelvic control. If we don't have good pelvic control, we can't expect our walking to be as comfortable or efficient as we'd like. The fact is, many people have lost control of the position of their pelvis without knowing it. This can be a common cause of walking problems, hip problems and even a significant contributor to back pain.[11]

So, how can you tell if you've got a problem with controlling your pelvis? One easy way is to try to move your pelvis and take note of how easy (or difficult) it may be. To do this, start off standing with your hands on your hips. Without moving your lower back or your knees, can you roll your pelvis forward, sticking your bottom out? And now can you roll your pelvis backward, tucking your tailbone between your legs and pulling your bottom in? You can see images of these movements on page 127 (*top*).

If these movements seem foreign or difficult to you, there's a high probability that your pelvic control isn't up to scratch.

Many people can do one of these pelvic movements but not the other. If this is the case, it's likely that certain muscles have shortened over time and you are favoring one of these tilted pelvic positions when you stand and walk.

There are many ways to correct this, but working on rolling the pelvis forward and backward from a variety of positions is a great place to start. You might want to spend a few minutes every day practising the cat–cow exercise below as a great way to start rebuilding some pelvic control.

Once you feel that you've "loosened up" your stiff pelvis, you may notice that your back, hip and knee troubles are much easier. You may notice that you can walk further than before and that you tire less easily. All of these positive effects can come from just a few minutes per day of practising the following movement.

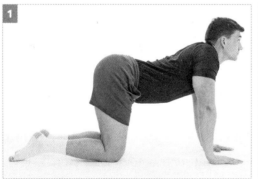 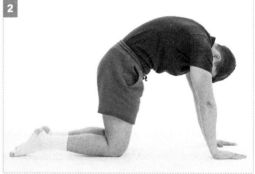

Start on all fours, either on a soft floor or on your bed. First, roll your pelvis forward and stick your bottom up in the air, allowing your back to form a 'U' shape. Lift your head as you do this (1). Hold this position for two seconds, then proceed to invert it by arching your back and tucking your pelvis underneath you and dropping your head (2). Alternate between these two positions, holding each only for two seconds, for about 20 repetitions. Repeat three times a day.

"No Hands!"—The Key to Maintaining Strength and Balance Over Fifty

There is one thing that scares people of the older generation like nothing else. It strips people of their independence and can land them in hospital, sometimes for days on end. Some unfortunately never make it back out. If you hadn't guessed, I'm talking about falls.

A fall can be absolutely catastrophic; and older people suffer disproportionately to other age groups. Due to higher risks of osteoporosis (or brittle bones) in this age group, a fall can be devastating. All it takes is one unfortunate landing to cause a fractured hip, broken wrist, or dislocated shoulder. Any of these injuries can cause significant disability and pain, for a very long time in some cases. It is for this reason that the NHS estimates falls cost the health service roughly £2 billion every year in the UK.[12] During my time working in my clinic, I have seen hundreds of patients following a fall that has led to significant injury, many of whom are still struggling months later. Most of these people did eventually recover, but many have experienced long-term effects on their quality of life resulting from that one fall.

I've also seen the aftermath of falls in my own family—with my grandmother suffering both a fractured hip and a fractured wrist from one fall at home. For me, that alone has been motivation enough to try to help whoever I can to avoid these terrifying falls. Older individuals fall for many reasons and sometimes these are unavoidable. However, two of the most common reasons for falling in people over fifty are poor balance and a loss of strength in the legs.[13]

As we grow older, we tend to lose some of our ability to balance. For a start, changes to the inner ear as we age lead to decreased ability to sense where the body is in space. The joints also become stiffer (often due to arthritis) and the muscles weaker (due to a process called sarcopenia) with advancing age. Lack of practice also plays a role: we tend to move less with age, and decreasing activity levels effectively mean we are more likely to be out of practice with walking around in general, leading to a loss of balance. Finally, eyesight can also be a factor, with older individuals being more likely to be visually impaired. Our eyesight is a key contributor to balance, so, if it loses some of its clarity, our balance suffers.

For these reasons, it would be unusual for someone to be able to stand on one leg at seventy as well as they could when they were thirty. But it is important to note that balance can be improved at just about any age. The human body has a clever way of becoming efficient at the things that we practice regularly. If we practice balancing just outside of our comfort zone from time to time, our balancing ability should improve.

To prove this point, sometimes I'll get a patient over fifty who comes into my office for a painful problem. When I test their balance, they have a phenomenal ability to stand on one leg. More often than not, when I marvel at how good they are (sometimes able to stand on one leg with their eyes closed), they smile and tell me about the yoga class they've attended every week for the past decade. These people rarely fall, even in older age. This proves that with regular practice, you can significantly improve your balance, even beyond seventy years of age.

While heading to find your nearest yoga class might be a good idea for many reading this, it isn't the only way to get the benefits I'm describing. There are some effective methods that can be put into action at home to improve your balance, starting today:

Practice Your Balance at Home

When practising balance tasks at home, you should always ensure your safety by starting off holding onto the kitchen worktop or the back of a chair until you find your feet. Never practice balance out of reach of something that you could quickly grab hold of to steady yourself if necessary. I recommend to my clients that they always start with the easiest variation of a balance exercise and build up. It should initially feel a little challenging but not impossible. Some good options for practising your balance include standing with your feet very close together and taking your fingers away from the worktop, one by one, as shown right:

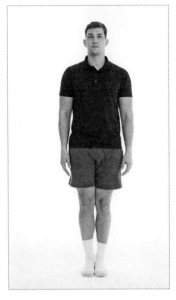

Close stance: note the feet touching and the narrow base of support.

Balance Progressions

If you can do this for 30 seconds with no bother, progress to a tandem stand with your feet in line, right heel touching left toes as if walking a tightrope. Make sure to swap legs after 30 seconds, then repeat, feet reversed. If you can do this for 30 seconds without feeling challenged at all, then try moving on to a single-leg stand. Both exercises are demonstrated on page 204.

I usually tell people to start holding onto the worktop with both hands, then take away their hand support, finger by finger. Once you feel steady and you've only got one finger on the worktop, try taking your hands off altogether. When you practice balancing in this way, be sure to always have someone nearby who can watch you and make sure that you're safe.

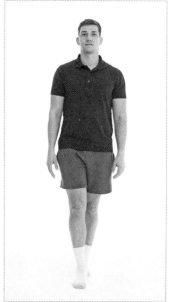 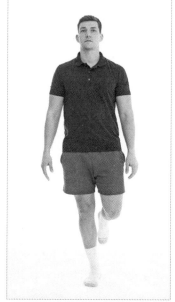

Position your feet one in front of the other, with the front heel touching the toes of the opposite foot. Try to hold this position for 30 seconds without wobbling.

Practice standing on one leg and maintaining your balance without wobbling. Aim for one minute each side.

Practice Getting Up and Out of a Chair

While your balancing ability is very important in avoiding falls, having significant strength in your lower limbs is crucial as well.[13] One of the simplest yet most effective ways of building and maintaining leg strength is by practising sitting down and standing up from a chair (*see next page*). Sit down as slowly as you possibly can (taking around four seconds to go from standing to sitting is good)—and here's the catch: using your hands is not allowed. If you practice this sit-to-stand movement daily, you're going to build significant strength in your hips and knees, safeguarding you from falls. Do not proceed with any exercise (including this one) if it is painful, and be sure to start from a higher chair (which should be easier) before trying this exercise from lower chairs.

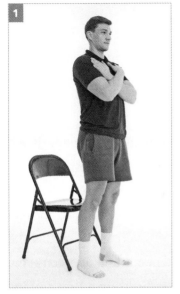 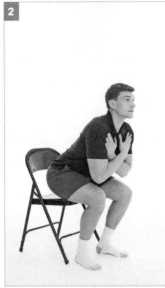

Start with the backs of your knees touching a firm chair (1). Taking a minimum of four seconds, slowly lower yourself to a sitting position (2). Stand up from the chair at normal pace, without the use of your hands, and repeat five times. Do this several times a day.

Working on your balance takes time: don't expect to see a huge improvement in the first few weeks. As with anything worth having, progress takes effort and plenty of consistent practice. However, I've yet to meet someone who tells me that avoiding a fractured hip and maintaining their independence in later life isn't worth a little hard work!

The Truth about Knee Arthritis

For many people over fifty, chances are that they can't get 10 minutes into a conversation with a group of close friends before someone brings up an ache, pain, or even surgery that they've had because of arthritis.

Arthritis is generally approached with an air of doom and gloom. After all, there's no denying that it is a leading cause of suffering, particularly in the Western world. The suffering caused by arthritis is also weaponized against us. The press often use poorly designed research studies to gain clicks with headlines that read something like "The Newest Arthritis Wonder Cure!" . . . only for us to read several lines in, that the dubious study being quoted found there was only a slight, tenuous link between some household ingredient or spice and minor pain relief from arthritis, in a tiny, specific subset of people that may or may not be statistically significant. The same is true of supplement companies, who frequently make claims about their products that hardly ever live up to the hype (more on supplements for arthritis later).

But what does it really mean to have arthritis? Is it a life sentence of pain, misery and suffering?

Although I cannot yet speak from lived experience, based on the improvements I see with my patients I would argue that it is doesn't have to be.

Arthritis, in medical terms, is the deterioration of the cartilage in a joint due to the process of aging. However, how this loss of cartilage is experienced differs dramatically from person to person.

You might assume that when your cartilage starts to deteriorate, your joints automatically become stiff and extremely painful, in direct proportion to the level of deterioration. This is not necessarily true. In recent studies where people over fifty have been put through an MRI scanner, the results show that almost everyone suffers from some degree of arthritis.[14] However, somewhat surprisingly, only a fraction of these people report any pain at all.

I have had too many clients to count who have come to see me for an entirely separate painful problem, only to have a scan done that picked up an incidental finding of severe arthritis in another area of the body—an area that has never given them any trouble whatsoever.

How can this be? How can some people suffer so badly, while others seem to get away with it, remaining free of symptoms their whole lives?

The short answer is, we don't fully understand the answer to this question yet—although we do have some clues as to what factors might contribute to the development of pain. For example, if you are overweight and there's more pressure traveling through an arthritic joint, it would make sense that this would lead to pain in some cases.[15]

Movement quality also has an impact. One other thing that has become clear to me during my years of practice is that if you take two people, one with stiff joints and the other with no stiffness, the one with the stiffness tends to suffer with worse pain than the one who has better movement, even if the degree of arthritis in that joint is the same in both people.[16]

This is certainly the case when we talk about knees. When someone comes to me for treatment of their knee arthritis, I always look at whether they can fully bend and straighten their knee. If they can't, that's the first thing I look to restore for them, and more often than not, it improves their symptoms reasonably quickly.

One thing I try to help people avoid, in my work as a physiotherapist, is the need to go under the knife for a total knee replacement. Most of my clients value living without the fear of risky surgery and I work toward helping them achieve that goal. While there's no denying the operations that orthopedic surgeons perform on people's knees are nothing short of incredible these days, at the time of writing, even the best total knee replacement will only last 10 to 15 years at most before it needs "revising." These revisions are never as straightforward as the first time around, so delaying surgery for as long as possible is vital.

Even after your first total knee-replacement surgery, the recovery process can be long and painful. It's a significant, major surgery; it should never be taken lightly. Total knee-replacement surgery can be risky and I always maintain that it should be a last resort.

If you can feel the rumblings of knee arthritis, which usually starts as a dull ache around the margins of your knee joint, there are some things you can do to ease the pain and improve your mobility without having to resort to surgery or reach for the painkillers:

Try to Maintain a Full Range of Movement at Your Knee Joint

If you struggle to press the back of your knee down into the bed when you're lying on your back, or you're unable to bend your knee fully so your heel almost touches your bottom, you've currently got a stiff knee joint. Stiff knees are often painful, but when this problem is corrected, symptoms usually improve to a degree, regardless of the underlying arthritis still remaining. You could practice gently bending and straightening your knee for several minutes each day to build some flexibility back into the knee joint (*demonstrated on page 183*). Over a number of weeks, you should notice a difference on stairs and getting into and out of chairs.

Use a Warm Compress on the Knee in the Morning

If you suffer like many others with morning stiffness in your knee for the first 15 minutes or so after getting out of bed, the first thing you should do as part of your morning routine is make a hot water bottle. By warming up the knee joint with a hot water bottle or hot bath, you can start to relieve stiffness and pain far quicker than if you wait for the area to "heat up" naturally. You can also use this method at other times when you notice stiffness and pain, which may be more common in the winter months.

Keep Active, Keep Walking

When in pain, staying active can be difficult, especially when the alternative is sitting by the fire with your feet up. However, continuing to walk regularly is especially important for those with arthritis. One reason for this is that having weak knee muscles contributes to the pain when there's some wear to the cartilage in your knees. Researchers from Korea University in Seoul found that those with less leg muscle experienced worse pain with knee arthritis.[17] By walking regularly, you can minimize the rate of muscle loss in your legs and keep those knee joints well protected. The old adage "if you don't use it, you lose it" is very true when it comes to the strength that can be maintained with walking. It won't be long before disuse leads to lack of ability to go on those long hikes, sometimes permanently if you're not careful. Keep active, keep walking, and keep those legs as strong as you can.

Ask Your Doctor about Capsaicin Cream

Capsaicin cream is a reasonably new product in Western medicine, but its arthritis-relieving qualities have been known about in the Far East for many centuries. Capsaicin is one of the substances in chilli peppers that gives them their heat, and applying this substance in the form of a cream to the skin over an arthritic joint has been shown to provide effective relief for many people.[18] Capsaicin cream is, unfortunately, a prescription-only medicine in the UK at the time of writing, and may not be suitable for all, but if you ask your doctor for some they are usually happy to oblige.

The Truth about Hip Arthritis

The fact that arthritis can be present even in the absence of pain is as true when it comes to your hips as it is with your knees. However, pain from hip arthritis can be truly debilitating for many people, significantly impacting their quality of life.

Hip arthritis usually shows up as pain in the groin rather than on the outside of the hip, although the latter can occasionally occur. You might feel a restriction to movement at your hip joint, or notice more clicking and clunking than usual. Walking in hilly areas may become more challenging. In the later stages of hip arthritis, some people report a scary sensation of "giving way" at the hip, as if their muscles suddenly refuse to support them any longer.

In terms of treatment, the same principles apply for hip arthritis as for knee arthritis: remaining strong in the surrounding muscles and keeping your capacity for movement is key, echoed in a recent review on the topic of hip arthritis.[19] From my experience, I have observed that hips can be protected from many of the nasty symptoms of arthritis by maintaining a good range of motion.

What does a good range of motion in the hips look like? Well, for a start, you should be able to put your socks on and take them off without too much trouble. You should also be able to get in and out of a low car seat without feeling stiffness or tightness in your hip or groin.

If you struggle with either of these daily tasks, it's a good idea to arrange to see someone who can help you improve the movement in your hips as quickly as you possibly can, to prevent the problem from progressing any further. This may come as a surprise, but even if you've started to lose mobility in your hips, it isn't necessarily the start of a downward spiral into declining mobility—provided you do something about it early. Through certain hands-on methods (such as Mulligan mobilizations), physiotherapists have developed ways to help their clients improve hip mobility and maintain good hip health, despite the effects of aging, while exercises also help.

The other incredibly useful approach we can take with people suffering from this condition is to help them strengthen the muscles that support the hip joint. This can "offload" the joint and help to stop that horrible "giving way" sensation. Below are a selection of my favorite hip-strengthening exercises that are often useful for those with hip arthritis:

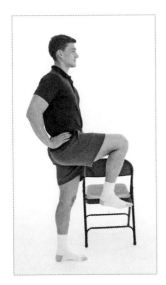 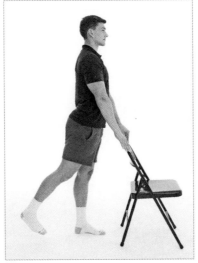 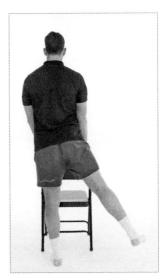

Start in a standing position. You can strengthen the hip in all planes of movement: flexion (left), extension (centre) and abduction (right). Repeat each of the movements above 10 to 15 times in a row, then move on to the next movement, several times a day.

One big difference that exists between hip and knee arthritis is what you can expect following joint-replacement surgery with the two conditions. Knee-replacement surgery is more complex and carries a longer recovery time (as well as possibly more pain and disability in the first six weeks after the operation), while hip-replacement surgery is usually simpler, with a smoother recovery. Either way, both are major surgeries and should always be regarded as such.

At my clinic, we have many health-conscious clients who are admirably determined to take their health into their own hands, refusing to rely on medical procedures as a means for "fixing" age-related aches and pains. The results we achieve with some of these clients are amazing and show the potential for improvement in hip arthritis without necessarily needing to undergo risky surgery. My advice for most people is the same: do everything you can to make the most of the hip or knee joint you already have before opting for a replacement.

The Single Best
Hip and Knee Exercise

While most of my clients value their health greatly, they also value anything that is going to save them time and unnecessary energy. By the time you reach the age of fifty, you've probably come to the realization that your time is far too precious to waste on things that aren't adding value to your life.

That's why, when it comes to health and my approach with my clients, I always prioritize strategies, tips and exercises that are going to give my clients the greatest "bang for their buck" from a time perspective. Less is often more. People are surprised to learn that I often only give my clients one carefully selected exercise to begin rehabilitation. So, for this section, I thought I'd show you the single most valuable exercise (in my humble opinion) you can do for your hips and knees, to maintain strength and function throughout the rest of your life.

We call this exercise the "goblet squat" and I've chosen it for its practicality, ease of use and the incredible benefits it provides.

The goblet squat falls into the category of a "compound exercise": one that uses multiple joints and muscle groups. We perform some variation of the goblet squat most days without even realizing it. Simply getting up and out of a chair without using your hands is the starting variation of the goblet squat, and is the place I recommend most people start. But once you are strong enough to manage it, adding external load is a great way to get stronger.

As with all the exercises in this book, the goblet squat exercise won't be suitable for everyone; avoid it if it causes you pain.

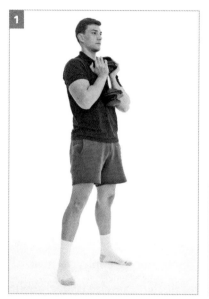 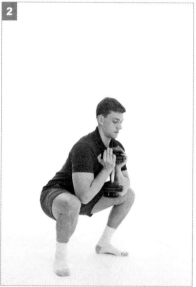

Start by holding a weight or a bag of books close to your chest (1). Keeping your back straight, bend at the hips and knees as if to sit back. Slowly sink down as low as you can comfortably (2) – never into pain – then stand back up again. Complete 10 to 15 repetitions of this exercise, rest for a minute, then repeat two or three times.

Once you can do more than 15 repetitions with ease, find something a little heavier to hold.

To perform this exercise correctly, you need to hinge at both the hips and the knees. The two muscle groups responsible for controlling this hinging action are the muscles in the buttock area (called the gluteal muscles or glutes) and the muscles at the front of the thigh (called the quadriceps). These are the main muscles that allow us to walk and stand without our knees or hips giving way. Therefore, by strengthening them further, we improve every activity that involves standing or being on our feet (i.e. almost everything!).

You'll also see in the pictures that a small weight is held in front, near to the chest. This is what gives the exercise the name "goblet squat," because it involves holding a dumbbell as if it were a goblet in front of the body (an old-fashioned term, granted). By holding a dumbbell, you're adding some extra resistance, which challenges the hip and knee muscles further and builds strength more than just performing the exercise with your body weight. However, you may need to start with just your body weight in order to get going, then progress from there.

To make this exercise easier or harder, you can choose whether or not your bottom makes contact with a seat when you drop down to the lowest point. If you make contact with a seat, it will take the tension off the muscles for a while and should make the exercise easier, in theory. However, in practice, this also takes away momentum from your movement and may actually make it feel harder (as you'll be standing up from the chair from a completely still start). Either way, the exercise works fabulously for improving your mobility and strength, and translates well to many activities we perform every day without thinking, such as walking, getting in and out of a car, climbing stairs and picking things up from the floor.

I always recommend working in a pain-free range and building up from there, trying to increase the depth of the squat as time goes on and movement becomes more comfortable. You don't need to start off going as low as the image shows. Starting off by dipping down just 15cm (6in) is often enough for those who are carrying an injury.

Start by performing a set of 5 to 10 repetitions and then build up to 15 repetitions in a row. If you can do 15 with no problem, find something slightly heavier to hold in front of you (you do not necessarily need to go and invest in a set of dumbbells; a big book or a bag filled with something heavy would be a good starting point).

Pain on the Side of Your Hip? It's Probably *Not* Arthritis!

In my clinic at HT Physio, I regularly see people (especially women over fifty) who are suffering from pain at the side of their hip that just doesn't seem to get any better, no matter what they try.

A lot of people assume that this must be the first signs of hip arthritis rearing its ugly head. However, more often than not, this pain is caused by something else entirely.

Most cases of pain at the side of the hip are caused by an injury to the tendons around the side of the hip, or inflammation of a little fluid sac around this area called the bursa. This injury has a few different names, including gluteal tendinopathy or bursitis, an old-fashioned term. We used to try to tell these two problems apart, but we don't any longer (mostly because the gluteal tendons and bursa are almost always both affected). Instead, we recently gave this condition a new name: greater trochanteric pain syndrome (or GTPS).

GTPS is just a clever term for pain around the bony area on the side of your hip (called the greater trochanter). It is characterized by:

- Pain on the outside of the hip (that can sometimes radiate)

- Tenderness to touch around the side of your hip

- Pain when walking and standing

- Difficulty standing on one leg

- Pain walking up or down stairs

- Pain walking up or down hills

GTPS is a very common problem—in fact, research shows it will affect 10 to 25 percent of the population, making it as common as hip arthritis—and just as debilitating in many cases.[20]

We see it a lot more commonly in women than in men because of a difference in the shape of our pelvises. Women tend to have wider-set pelvises (think of the traditional "hourglass" shape of a woman's curves) than men, and this puts the tendons in the hip into a stretch that can predispose women to GTPS. Sorry, ladies!

A very subtle, long-standing weakness in the gluteal muscles that affects the way you walk or stand can lead to repetitive strain on the structures on the side of your hip. This repetitive strain leads to tiny tears in the tendons and inflammation in the little fluid sac (or bursa) on the side of your hip, which can lead to GTPS.

In most cases of this problem, weakness of the gluteal muscles precedes the start of pain.[21] Women require more gluteal muscle strength than men to walk properly (again, because of the differences in the way their pelvises are built), but most of the ladies I assess in clinic also have poor hip muscle strength. This leaves them at risk of problems like GTPS.

However, if you've developed pain on the side of your hip, it isn't too late to address the deficiency in your hip strength. In fact, restoring the strength of the hip muscles is actually one of the best ways to treat GTPS. There are also some absolutely must-know "rules" when it comes to this condition that, when followed, can dramatically improve your rate of recovery:

Get Comfortable

With GTPS, getting comfortable at night can be a challenge. If you're going to lie on your bad side at night, consider lying on top of a soft duvet which can "cushion" the area below your hip and prevent pressure from aggravating the injury.

Use a Pillow

If you're going to lie on your opposite side at night, be sure to place a pillow between your legs. This is important. Letting your legs cross over the midline of your body compresses the painful area (even when you don't directly feel pain from it) and can prevent the problem from getting better. Most of us are side-sleepers, so we run the risk of spending eight hours every night with our bad leg crossed over midline—not good for the hips! By placing a pillow between your legs, you can ensure the bad leg doesn't cross over the midline of the body, which should relieve some pressure from the painful area.

Don't "Hip Hang"!

Most of us are guilty of this, shifting from one foot to the other while standing, chatting away to a friend. The problem with this is that as we place all of our weight on one leg, our hips move over to one side, increasing pressure on the affected area as we "hang" by our hips. Again, this can aggravate GTPS, so make sure you stand with your weight spread evenly between your feet, at least until the painful problem settles down.

Stop Crossing Your Legs!

This might be the hardest habit to break, but it's incredibly important. When you cross your legs while sitting or even lying on your back, you put pressure through the painful area, aggravating the side of your hip. This is one of the biggest causes of the problem in the first place, and chronic leg-crossing definitely prevents a lot of people from getting better as fast as they should. Be sure to avoid crossing your legs—if necessary, ask a partner to remind you to uncross every time they see you do so.

Avoid Very Low Chairs

By sitting in low chairs, you're asking your hip muscles to work very hard to lift you back out of the chair. The pressure from this action can aggravate the problem and cause a lot of pain. Try placing a pillow under your bottom when sitting in the low chairs around your house to help yourself.

Don't Stand on One Leg

You may laugh at this one, but a lot of us do exactly that every day when we put on and take off our trousers, shoes, and socks! Make sure you get dressed while sitting whenever possible if you don't do so already.

Try to Avoid Extra-Long Walks or Going Up and Down Hills Where Possible

You may find that walking aggravates your hip pain and you struggle to walk as far as you once could. When suffering from GTPS, "no pain, no gain" is not a sensible approach. You should listen to what your hip is telling you: If it's painful, don't try to push through! Take a break and get back to your walk when it's settled again. Hills are probably the biggest challenge for people with this problem, so try to avoid steep hills where you can. Do try to keep active; however, you may benefit from temporarily cutting down your overall walking distance until the pain settles.

Use the Handrail Whenever Climbing Stairs

Stairs are another common daily activity that aggravates GTPS. Try to walk upstairs using the handrail, to take a bit of pressure off your hip.

There are certain targeted exercises that are extremely effective at improving the pain associated with GTPS. However, the technique has to be absolutely spot-on for these exercises to be effective, so you may want to get some supervision from a specialist before giving them a try. That said, the banded clam exercise below is the one I give to many of my clients with GTPS and is a great way to start the recovery process for many people:

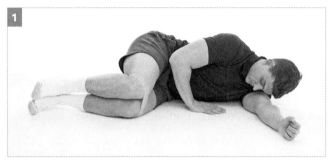

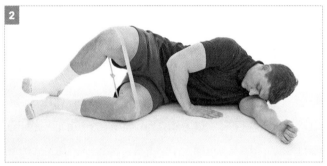

Lie on your side, with the side to be worked on top. Tie a resistance band around both thighs, just above the knees. Bend both knees, keeping your knees and ankles together (1). Without rolling backward, lift your top knee up toward the ceiling, stretching the band (2). Slowly return your knee to the start position and repeat, 10 to 15 times in a row, several times a day.

A more basic version of this exercise, without the band, can be found on page 166.

What to Do When Knee Pain Affects Your Walking

There are likely to be many people reading this section who have knee problems which stop them from walking as far as they'd like. When knee pain limits walking, it can affect your life, not just on a physical level, but on a social level as well. Walking is a hobby that can be enjoyed with friends and loved ones. When this is threatened, those socializing opportunities are threatened as well.

This section is designed to provide recommended steps to take if you find yourself in a position where your walks have become less comfortable, or you aren't able to go as far as you'd like because of your knee pain.

My first piece of advice to the people I talk with is to tell them to get checked out, so they know exactly what's causing their knee pain. However, as I have mentioned several times in this book, this doesn't necessarily mean that getting an X-ray or MRI scan is the best option. The causes of most knee pain can be diagnosed clinically, either by a physiotherapist or a doctor with experience in assessing knees. There are very subtle differences in signs and symptoms between the causes of knee pain which can easily be missed, so it's important to get assessed by a specialist.

Once you know what's going on, you can formulate a treatment plan designed around your goals and current levels of fitness. If your goal is to walk 20 miles each week, your treatment program should look different to someone whose goal is simply to be able to climb the stairs without pain. If you feel you've been given a generic, one-size-fits-all treatment plan, you should seek a better, more personalized alternative.

Your goals will also dictate the time it takes to achieve an acceptable outcome. If you just want to achieve some degree of pain relief, this can usually be done with a few treatment sessions, over the course of several weeks. However, in order to fix the underlying problem and ensure that your knees stay healthy for years to come, a greater investment of time will be needed.

Other than having one-on-one treatment, if knee pain is affecting your walking, there are a few things you can do that will improve things:

Experiment with a Knee Brace

While knee supports don't "fix" the underlying problem, they might just help you complete that long walk without being forced to stop. There is conflicting evidence about whether they help to prevent twists and sprains, but I figure they are unlikely to do harm, so may be worth considering.[22]

Try a Walking Pole

Almost all of my clients hate the idea of using a walking stick (and the desire to walk independently without needing to use a stick any longer is a common reason my clients approach me in the first place), but using a walking pole for long hikes affords you the support of a stick without the stigma attached to a true "walking aid." Walking poles are regularly used by all members of the walking community, regardless of age or knee health and, anecdotally, reduce knee discomfort on long walks (despite research showing little to no effect on actual walking mechanics[23]), as well as possibly improving endurance, too. They can be picked up relatively inexpensively from a variety of outdoor or sports stores and are growing in popularity as each year passes. You can find a video I recorded demonstrating how to use walking poles in Video D in the Resources section (*see page 413*).

Keep Your Knees Warm, Especially in Winter

If you ever feel like you start off stiff for the first 15 minutes of a walk but then "loosen up" as the walk goes on, you'll probably benefit from pre-warming your knees before any kind of walk, as well as keeping your knees warm as you continue. This may involve really blasting the car heater before you start your walk, as well as wearing long johns or leggings for winter walks. Many of my clients are truly surprised at the difference this tip makes. Letting a sore joint become cold is a sure-fire route to discomfort, so try to avoid it where possible.

If Pain Continues, Try Cycling for a While

Most of my clients with knee pain while walking actually find cycling to be a pain-free activity. Cycling is as good, if not better, for building and maintaining cardiovascular fitness and good heart health. You'll also find that it places significantly less stress on your knees than walking or jogging. It can be a good temporary alternative for those struggling with walking.

Build Some Strength in the Swimming Pool

The true conundrum faced by many people with knee pain is that they need to get their legs strong to improve their symptoms—but their knee pain stops them from exercising effectively to become stronger. As a solution to this problem, I often recommend my clients start a strengthening routine in the swimming pool. The water immediately takes 50 percent of your body weight away from your lower limbs, which is usually enough to diminish any of the usual pain felt while walking on land. Walking in the water is usually a pain-free way of improving your strength (both on land and in the water) that can work wonders for people with knee pain. Start off by walking a few widths in the water, striding out against the resistance of the water in the pool. You'll find yourself getting tired quicker than you would walking on land (which is a good thing). One more thing: if you choose to swim, be careful with breast stroke. For many people with knee pain, swimming breast stroke can aggravate the problem. Stick to breast-stroke arms and front-crawl legs instead.

Strengthen the Key Muscles

Many people who suffer with knee pain when walking are victims of poor muscular control around the knee and lower limb, leading to excess stress on the knee joint during gait. The solution to this problem is to improve knee and hip muscle strength. Two exercises to combat this problem are the straight-leg raise and side-lying hip abductions, shown on pages 195 and 166 (*bottom*), respectively.

Stretch the Calves

Another common cause of knee pain when walking is tightness in the surrounding muscles. One muscle group in particular can lead to knee pain when tight: the calf. Formed of three different muscles, the calf muscle primarily controls movement at the ankle—but it has a strong influence on the knee as well. As the calf muscle crosses over the knee joint, when it becomes tight it can compress the structures within the knee

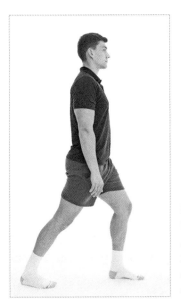

and cause stress on the joint, especially when walking. Thankfully, stretching the calf muscle is easy and can be a great solution. If it is comfortable for you to do so, try the gentle calf stretch exercise shown left to improve the flexibility of this key muscle:

Put the leg to be stretched behind you, keeping the heel down on the floor. Keeping the back leg straight, bend the front knee until you feel a stretch in your calf in the back leg. Hold this stretch for a minimum of 30 seconds, several times a day on each side. Stand with both hands on a wall or the back of a chair if you feel you need extra stability.

Catching in the Hip

We previously spoke about the fact that arthritis of the hip can cause groin pain. However, this is not the only common hip problem to affect over-fifties, causing pain in the groin.

I once met with a new patient who first came into my office absolutely devastated after being told by her doctor that she was suffering with arthritis in her hip. This lady was in her early fifties, very active and a member of about four different exercise classes (around which her social life revolved). She had reported "catching" and stiffness in the groin, which had developed over the last six months. Recognizing the stiffness and pain as a symptom of arthritis, the doctor had informed her she might one day need a hip replacement and should avoid some of her exercise classes. She came to me to see if there was a viable alternative.

Given this lady's history and the symptoms of her pain, it was possible that arthritis was the cause; but at her age and given the "catching" symptom she was experiencing, I suspected something different. The cause I suspected was a labrum tear.

The labrum is a thin layer of cartilage that sits around the rim of the hip joint. The hip is a ball-and-socket joint, meaning it fits together like a ball inside a socket, and the labrum enables the ball to fit more securely inside the hip socket. The problem with the labrum is that it is a soft tissue, and sometimes it can develop nicks and tears. As the ball rotates inside the socket, it can catch on a labrum tear, which brings about the common symptom of "catching" in the groin for people with this injury.

This injury tends to be most common in women over the age of fifty, affecting women more than men because the shape of their pelvis differs slightly. It is also common in the active population and people who attend yoga and Pilates classes, due to positions the hip is put into during these activities.

Thankfully, although they can take a long time to get better, labrum tears usually heal without the need for surgery. The key to treating these injuries is gentle strengthening and as much help as possible to improve pelvic control. I usually recommend my clients stop any aggressive stretching of the hip, as the extremes of motion can put stress on the labrum and delay healing. Gentle movement is beneficial, with range of motion exercises (within the realms of comfort) being useful. Walking is also a great exercise for people with labrum tears, although runners should be cautious.

As for my patient, we found a resolution to her problem within about six months of treatment. It took about three months to see any improvement whatsoever in her symptoms, but then changes started to slowly happen, continuing until she was pain-free. She is now back to enjoying all her active hobbies and is able to use the gym four times a week again. Alongside the modified clam exercise (*see page 145*), the single-leg dip (*below*) and the bridge (*next page*) are two of the exercises we used to help her rebuild pelvic control and promote healing:

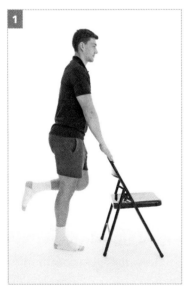 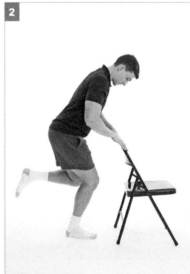

Support yourself on the back of a chair with both hands. Stand just on the leg to be worked (1). Bending at the hip and knee, dip down several inches, then come back up (2). Repeat 15 to 20 times in a row, several times a day.

Lying on your back with your knees bent, flatten your lower back into the bed or floor (1). Pushing through your heels, lift your pelvis until there is a straight line between your knees and shoulders. At the top of the movement, squeeze your buttocks and hold for a few moments (2). Slowly lower to the start position. Repeat 10 to 15 times, several times a day.

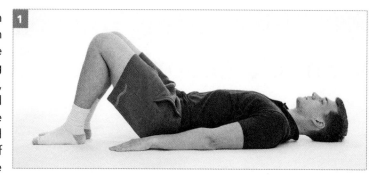

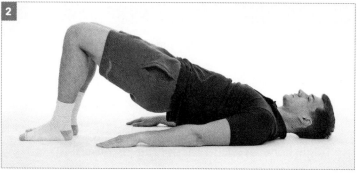

Protecting Your Natural Shock Absorber: the Meniscus

Inside our knees, there are two different types of cartilage that help the joint to function. The first is the hyaline cartilage, which lines the surfaces of the bones in the knee. This is the cartilage type associated with arthritis when it wears away.

The second type of cartilage is called the meniscus. The meniscus is made of fibrocartilage and acts more like a shock absorber, and it sits between the two main bones in the knee. Its job is to stop force transmitting up through the shin bone into the thigh bone. A well-functioning meniscus is your protective mechanism from unnecessary wear and tear over time.

The issue with the meniscus is that it can also degenerate over time as we age. It is very tightly attached to the tibia (shin bone), which means it cannot tolerate twisting, especially with a planted foot. As we age, the normally well-hydrated meniscus can dry out and become brittle. Over years of normal use, including twisting, the meniscus can develop tiny tears, which can progress into larger tears.

A meniscus tear feels a lot like arthritis for many people. Most of the time, the pain develops on the inside of the knee. There may be tenderness to touch along the joint line. It can sometimes cause a sensation of clicking, popping, or catching. In extreme cases, a meniscus tear can cause the knee to lock.

I treat painful meniscus tears very often at my clinic and the common factor between all of them is that they take a long time to get better. The reason for this is due to poor blood supply to the meniscus, which means healing is much slower than, say, a muscle tear. Suffering for over six months is not uncommon.

The changes we suffer to the meniscus are mostly unavoidable as we age—but there are some simple measures we can take to protect our little shock absorbers. Prevention is worth far more than cure, and avoiding a painful meniscus tear is a prize well worth the effort. Below are some simple tips to help you protect your meniscus (which may also help if you already have a meniscus injury):

Avoid Twisting

Our knees are designed to perform just two movements happily: bending and straightening. Twisting is not a particularly good movement for the knee as the meniscus has very little "give" in it in rotational movements. Try to avoid twisting with a planted foot, as this is the cause of many of the cases of a torn meniscus that I see.

Use Heat

If you are suffering from niggling knee pain over the joint line, using a hot compress on the affected area can be effective for bringing blood flow to the area and promoting healing.

Consider Ultrasound Treatment

I often use ultrasound treatment on an injured knee if I suspect a meniscus tear might be the cause. Ultrasound has been shown to promote healing in stubborn injuries and may help to speed up the process if the meniscus is injured.[24]

Maintain a Full Range of Motion

Keeping stiffness at bay is key for optimal knee health. Most people develop knee stiffness insidiously over time, because they don't make an effort to take their knee through a full range of motion regularly. A full range of motion keeps the structures inside the knee (including the meniscus) healthy, reducing the risk of problems later.

This can be achieved by lying on your back and bending the knee as much as possible, just to the point of stiffness, then straightening again, best performed little and often (*see page 183*).

Keep Strong

Having strong muscles surrounding and supporting the knee is essential. If one has weakness in the quadriceps in the thigh, and glutes in the hip, the knee is unprotected from stress and strain. This is one of the main causes of injury in the first place and can be prevented through regular exercise. I recommend the goblet squat exercise shown on page 214 as a great starting point.

Avoid Tight Calves

Tight calves lead to an increase in stress on the knee joint. Contrary to what most people think, the calves do not stop at the lower leg but actually have two attachments above the knee joint on the thigh bone. This means that tight calves compress the inner structures of the knee, which can lead to an increased risk of meniscus injury. You can stretch the calves effectively using the exercise on page 224.

Keep Moving

With or without a meniscus tear, walking is an essential exercise for almost everybody. It keeps the knee mobile and helps lubricate the joint. This can help prevent meniscus injuries and speed up healing for existing tears.

Sleep with a Pillow

Putting a plump pillow between the knees when lying on your side, or under the knees when lying on your back, can help prevent twisting of the knee during the night and settle an aggravated meniscus tear.

Hip and Knee Surgery Signs

Even with the perfect physiotherapy program, there are some sufferers of hip and knee arthritis whose symptoms will continue to progress until they have no choice but to consider surgery. While I am an advocate for doing everything possible to avoid surgery, there are some instances where I will refer a patient on for an orthopedic opinion. Below are some of the signs I look for that might indicate a person is an appropriate candidate for hip or knee surgery:

Hip and Knee Signs

- **No improvement, despite physio treatment:** This is the big one and I would almost never refer someone on for a surgical opinion without at least trying to achieve an improvement in their symptoms. If you have had a considerable (i.e. three months) course of treatment, including hands-on therapy and exercise, but there has been no improvement, an onward referral might be a good idea.

- **Unable to walk more than 100 yards (approx. 90m):** If you are unable to walk further than 100 yards comfortably, this is a sign the joint is lacking integrity and may need replacing.

- **Night pain:** If you are kept awake at night by the pain and your sleep is considerably disturbed, it makes sense to consider an orthopedic opinion—it doesn't take long for sleep deprivation to begin to cause other problems.

- **Relying on painkillers:** If you can't get through your day without painkillers, despite treatment from a physiotherapist, it might be time to consider a surgical opinion.

- **Dangerous "giving way":** The hip or the knee giving way is a common symptom in people with arthritis but it can often be cured by strengthening exercises, such as the goblet squat on page 214. However, if you are suffering with giving way of the hip or the knee that continues despite strengthening exercise, it could be a degenerated joint causing it (rather than simply weakness in the surrounding muscles).

Hip-Specific Signs

- **Shoes and socks:** If you are unable to independently put on and take off your shoes and socks, despite treatment from a physio, your arthritis may have progressed to the point where you have very little rotation of the hip. This can be a sign a surgical opinion is a good idea.

- **Car and bath:** If you can't get in and out of the bath or the car without assistance, this is another sign your hip is not happy.

- **Unable to sit:** In severe cases of hip arthritis, a sufferer might lose so much hip flexion they are unable to sit in a position where their hip is bent to 90 degrees. If this is the case and it doesn't respond to physio treatment, it might be time to consider your options.

Knee-Specific Signs

- **Unable to bend more than 90 degrees (despite treatment):** If your knee is not able to bend to more than 90 degrees, there are many cases where hands-on physiotherapy can significantly increase your range of motion. I saw a man in my clinic who originally came in with only 80 degrees of flexion, meaning he could not squat, kneel, or even climb stairs properly. Within about four weeks, his knee flexion was up to 130 degrees, unlocking all of these previously impossible activities. However, if you have had treatment and your knee is still so stiff you cannot bend it more than 90 degrees, it might be worth getting a second opinion.

- **Visible change in shape:** If your knee bows outward (called varus) or drops inward (*called valgus, see pages 236–237*), this might be because of structural changes within the joint. These changes in shape cannot usually be solved with physio, so might need looking at by a surgeon if they are causing you pain.

- **Locking:** Some knee injuries cause a strange and unpleasant symptom called "locking," which is where the knee gets stuck in one position and has to be manipulated to free it up. This usually happens when the knee is straight and it can be alarming to the sufferer. Persistent locking may mean something (like the meniscus) is trapped within the joint. A surgical opinion is often recommended for these instances.

Despite my recommendations against surgery for most people, in the modern day hip and knee operations are successful in the overwhelming majority of cases. If you do need surgery, don't panic! The key is to not opt for surgery before you've exhausted your other options—and find a surgeon you trust.

How to Strengthen Your Knees to Prevent "Giving Way"

Have you ever been out for a walk and noticed your knee feeling like it might buckle under you? If so, you have experienced what we call "giving way."

Giving way is a common symptom of many different knee problems. The quadriceps (or quads for short) are the muscles of the thigh above the knee joint that are responsible for keeping your knee straight when you stand and walk. Giving way is caused by the quads momentarily "cutting out" or being unable to support the knee due to weakness. Once the quads are out of action, there is nothing left to support the knee joint and the knee buckles. Most times, the quads can switch on again in time to catch you. But in serious cases, giving way can lead to a fall—with often devastating consequences.

Injuries and pain can cause the quads to cut out due to something called "muscle inhibition." This is one of the symptoms of an injury or painful problem, and happens when the brain registers that there is a problem with a joint. In response, it tries to shut down the surrounding muscles to protect the injured area. Unfortunately, this is an unhelpful response in most cases and leads to an acute loss of strength in the area, causing the knee to give way if it crosses a certain threshold.

Giving way can also be caused by a loss of muscle mass and strength, which develops over time due to deconditioning after an injury or due to arthritis. With pain in the knee joint, one tends to do less exercise over time, leading to a loss of muscle size and strength. This weakness can often first become noticeable when the knee gives way on a walk or coming down stairs.

Thankfully, in most cases, giving way of the knee is a fixable problem, even if the underlying arthritis or injury remains. The priority is to strengthen the quad muscles surrounding the knee joint in a way that is neither painful nor aggravating to an inflamed knee. Below are references to my favorite exercises for strengthening weak quad muscles and preventing giving way (only stick with an exercise if it is pain-free):

- Straight-leg raise exercise on page 195 (*top*).

- Inner-range quads exercise on page 195 (*bottom*).

- Single-leg dip exercise on page 226.

Reduce Knee Pain
with "Priming"

When it comes to knee pain, there is one important muscle that is the cause of much suffering, despite—or, perhaps, because of—getting little attention from most people. The reason this muscle gets away with the trouble it causes with knees is because it sits nowhere near the knee. Its name is the *gluteus medius*.

The gluteus medius (*covered in more detail on pages 163–166*) is a muscle of the hip. Its job is to keep the thigh bone (femur) straight when we walk and stand. The problem with the gluteus medius is that it is often weak in people who lead Western lives. Daily sitting, poor posture and lack of exercise all contribute to weakness in the gluteus medius, which usually goes unnoticed due to other muscles' ability to compensate. However, when the gluteus medius becomes weak, the femur cannot align properly and we experience something called valgus.

Valgus occurs when the thigh bone tracks at an inward angle, as opposed to directly down toward the ground. This puts undue stress on the inside of the knee and can be a contributing factor in a lot of knee pain. It is possible to have permanent valgus (which is a type of deformity of the knee) or functional valgus, which means the bones are straight but the knee falls inward during movement.

You can often tell whether you have an element of functional knee valgus by what happens when you descend stairs. Get a friend to watch you coming down stairs and ask them if your weight-bearing knee slightly rolls inward. If it does, it could be a sign of weakness in the glutes.

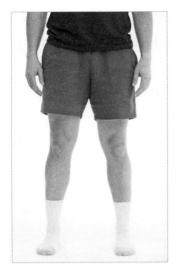

Normal knees

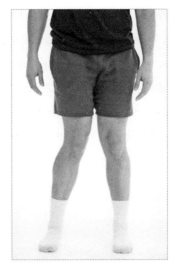

Valgus: note how the right knee turns inward toward the midline of the body

If you are suffering with functional valgus, don't panic! It is usually treatable through strengthening exercises over the long term. However, the same strengthening exercises that fix it over the long term can also bring about short-term benefits, too.

Every time we activate a muscle that has a poor mind–muscle connection, we not only improve that connection over the long term but also give it a short-term boost. This is why some people find their knee instantly becomes less painful in the minutes after performing a set of glute-strengthening exercises; they haven't gained strength or muscle mass in the space of two minutes, but they have temporarily strengthened the mind–muscle connection to the muscle by "switching it on." I call this type of exercise pre-activation, or priming.

Priming exercises are designed to be done immediately before you are setting off for a walk, run, or cycle ride—or indeed just before any activity that would usually cause you discomfort. The goal of priming is to activate a muscle with poor connection, which increases the connection during the impending longer bout of exercise. Priming is perfect for waking up "lazy glutes," helping them to activate as they were designed to when you leave the house.

Below is a priming exercise I commonly recommend to my clients. This standing hip abduction with band exercise should be done with strict technique so as only to use the gluteal muscles. It should be performed until there is at least a little tiredness in the target muscle at the back of the hip, but never to the point of pain. The closer you can do it to the start of your longer bout of exercise, the better. The same exercise can be used regularly to build, not just connection, but permanent strength in the target muscles.

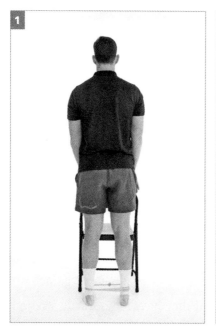
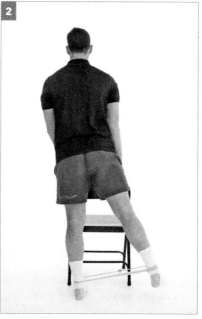

Start by standing with a resistance band around both ankles, holding on to a worktop or chair for support (1). Take all your weight onto just one leg. Keeping your spine perfectly straight, take your other leg out to the side and very slightly behind you in a diagonal motion (2). Slowly bring the leg back to the starting position and repeat on the same leg for about 10 to 15 times, for several sets just before you start the rest of your exercise session.

Part Six

FEET
AND
ANKLES

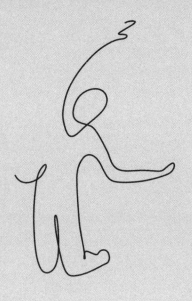

Introduction

Your feet aren't just the parts of your body that you may have lost the ability to reach down and touch several years ago. They are far more important than that. Like the tires of a car, they connect you to the ground and allow you to stand, walk and run with, hopefully, minimal difficulty.

But things can go wrong with our feet and ankles. When things do go wrong in these key areas, it often doesn't take long before we start to suffer in other parts of the body, too. Foot problems can lead to ankle problems, which lead to knee problems, which lead to problems with the back and the hips. Did you think that the toe pain with which you're currently suffering is only affecting that one tiny part of your body? Think again!

This basic fact about why our feet and ankles are so important isn't designed to scare you, though. I want to show you that you have a great opportunity to improve a small, responsive area of your body and bring about noticeable, positive changes elsewhere. We can help to ease knee arthritis simply by choosing the right footwear, for example. We can prevent a multitude of lower-limb problems by stretching one muscle group around the ankle. You may even be able to stop back pain . . . by massaging your feet!

In this chapter, you'll learn some techniques for preventing the common foot and ankle issues we help people with in my clinic. You'll also learn how to connect to your feet again; something we rapidly lose the ability to do in modern society. Pull your socks up and let's dip a toe into everything to do with the feet and ankles.

The Hidden Importance
of Ankle Mobility

I often look at the ankle and wonder at how such a small joint can have such an important role in the function of normal human movement. For a start, the ankle is the smallest of the three major lower-limb weight-bearing joints (hip and knee being the other two). It is a multidirectional joint, and when you combine that fact with its small size, this makes the ankle an inherently unstable joint. The design of the body is rarely an accident, and some degree of instability in the ankle is necessary to allow us to adapt to uneven ground, push off from the floor to run, or to bend deeply into a squat.

Over the course of a lifetime, many of us will sprain an ankle at least once. As it has plenty of inward rotation (called inversion) available to it, the ankle is prone to "inversion sprains." These sprains can cause damage to the ligaments on the outside of the ankle and, after a particularly bad sprain, it is common for the ankle to fail to return to its previous level of stability.

Sprains and injuries picked up over many years can combine with decreasing physical activity and the natural aging process to cause something common in the people I treat: a loss of ankle mobility.

One of the key signs of loss of ankle mobility is a decrease in the range of ankle dorsiflexion, shown opposite.

Ankle dorsiflexion is the act of pulling our toes up toward the shin and it is arguably the most important of the four ankle movements for normal activity.

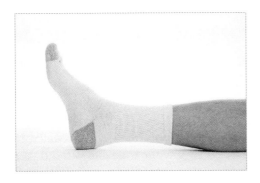

Normal resting ankle position.

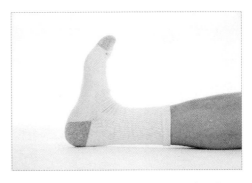

Ankle dorsiflexion: the action of pulling the toes up toward the shin.

For a start, when we walk, we need ankle dorsiflexion to allow the heel to strike the ground, then to allow the knee to pass over the toes later in our stride. Without this key movement, another area of the body must compensate: usually the knee or the hip. This loss of ankle mobility can lead to pain and injury in the knee or hip over time.

Second, we need good dorsiflexion to squat. We perform some kind of squat movement multiple times per day: sitting in a chair, getting off the toilet and bending down to pick something up all require some variation of a squat. During a normal squatting movement, the knee should travel over the toes and the only way it can do this is by using ankle dorsiflexion. If we lose this vital movement, once again, something else has to compensate and squatting suddenly becomes an injury risk to the knees, hips, or lower back.

So, how can you tell if you have lost ankle dorsiflexion? There is a simple knee-to-wall test (*see page 244 top*) you can do at home to reveal the answer.

If you did the test and found you couldn't get at least a 15cm (6in) gap between your toes and the wall while keeping your heel on the ground, it would be well worth addressing your loss of ankle mobility using the tips in this section. There's likely to be at least one of two causes for your loss of ankle mobility: muscle tightness or joint stiffness. There are a couple of simple exercises that can help you to regain lost dorsiflexion over time

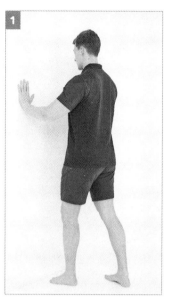 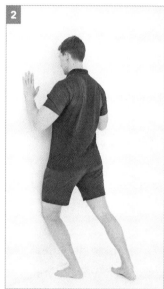

Position yourself facing a wall, with the leg to be tested planted with the toes just 15cm (6in) away from the wall (1). Keeping the heel of this foot on the ground, bend the knee and see if you can touch the wall with your knee cap without your heel lifting up (2). Picture 2 shows a 'pass' of this test. A 'fail' occurs when the heel lifts from the ground before the knee touches the wall.

to improve your walking, squatting, and general movement. The first great exercise to remedy this problem is the calf stretch (*see page 224*). The second exercise that can help is the chair-ankle mobilization (*below*):

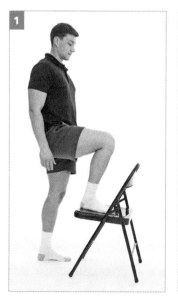 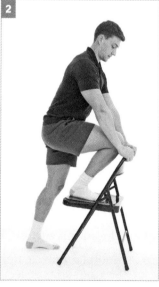

Stand facing a chair, with the foot of the side to be worked resting on the chair (1). Keeping the bottom of your heel in contact with the chair seat, bend the knee and bring your body weight over the top of the foot, until you feel a stretch in your ankle (2). Hold for just a few seconds then return to the start position. Repeat this action in a rhythmical way, two seconds out and two seconds in, for a total of one to two minutes, several times a day.

Stop Achilles Tendon
Pain in Its Tracks

Do you remember classical history lessons at school? The legend of the great Greek warrior Achilles was one of my favorite stories.

The legend has it that he was invincible, the greatest fighter ancient Greece had ever seen. His skill played a major part in the conquering of Troy, a so-called impenetrable city. The story goes that he was eventually felled in battle by an arrow that struck him through his heel, the first significant—and ultimately catastrophic—injury anyone had inflicted on him across any of the battles he had fought.

The legend of Achilles has been preserved by scholars of anatomy, who dubbed the large tendon joining the calf muscle to the heel the Achilles tendon. You can find your Achilles tendon at the back of your calf, just above the heel. It feels like a tough rope that you can easily grasp with two fingers. It is the largest tendon in the human body (a tendon joins muscle to bone) and it allows our calf muscles to pull on the heel and propel us onto our tiptoes.

However, a great many people suffer from a problem with the Achilles tendon, which can do a very good job of stopping active individuals in their tracks.[1] Achilles tendon pain usually starts as a niggle felt in the tendon itself or immediately beneath it, right on the heel bone. It often flares up during the first few minutes of walking and in the morning, then settles as you get warm. In more severe cases, it can be painful literally all the time that you're on your feet and can significantly affect walking and running for many people.

We call Achilles tendon pain "Achilles tendinopathy" (you might have heard of the term "Achilles tendinitis," which is an old-fashioned term for exactly the same thing).

This term basically means that there's a problem with the tendon or the area where the tendon attaches to the bone. The pain seems to be caused by inflammation, tiny little tears in the tendon, or the tendon holding onto too much water. All of these issues lead to the same result: a nagging pain at the back of the heel.

Luckily, unlike the injury suffered by our hero Achilles, this type of pain at the back of the heel is usually curable. If Achilles tendon pain has just started for you, our usual advice would be to rest for a couple of days and avoid any long walks or runs if possible. Usually, the pain will pass within three days.

However, if the pain has continued for longer than three days, a different approach is needed. Achilles tendon pain is usually preceded by a lack of strength in the calf muscles, which often goes undetected for many years, and can lead to excessive strain on the tendon.[2] When I say "lack of strength," what I'm really referring to is a lack of strength in relation to the demands you're asking of the tendon. For example, my Achilles tendon is strong enough for me to walk five miles or for me to work out in the gym for an hour without any bother at all, because I do those things regularly. However, if you asked me to run a marathon tomorrow, I'd be putting my Achilles tendon (and many other areas of my body) under intense pressure, something that it isn't used to.

This is a classic scenario for Achilles tendon pain. We often see it in people who go from being largely sedentary to suddenly deciding to take up an intense activity (we call these people the "weekend warriors"). This is one of the dangers of deciding to start out on a workout program like "Couch to 5K," where the participants are encouraged to start running and build up rapidly to five kilometers (three miles) of running distance. The Achilles tendon does not cope well with sudden changes in activity levels—and it may punish you for defying it.

A good general rule I tell my clients who are planning to increase their activity level is to only change one variable at a time (distance walked, duration of time walked or speed of walking) by a maximum of 10 percent at any one time. This is a great way to safeguard against Achilles tendon problems and many other injuries.

If you are already suffering from Achilles tendon pain, there are some steps you can take to reduce the pain and improve the health of the tendon that I'd like to share with you:

Be Careful When Stretching the Calves

One of the common Achilles pain myths tells us that if you have pain in your Achilles you should start stretching your calves immediately (*see page 224*). Unfortunately, this stretch has not necessarily been shown to improve Achilles tendon problems and holding this position for a long time may actually make the injury worse, especially if your pain is very close to the heel. Stretching the Achilles tendon can compress the injured part of the tendon and irritate the area, flaring it up and delaying healing.[3] While this effect doesn't occur for everyone, I think it's wise to resist the temptation to stretch the calf in the first instance.

Wear Supportive Shoes with a Heel

For a short period of time, it's advisable to wear sneakers and other shoes with a slightly raised heel wherever possible.[3] This will lift your heel up and take any stretch away from the Achilles tendon, allowing it to heal better for the reasons stated in the point above.

Try To Build Strength in Your Calves

One of the main causes of Achilles tendon problems is a mismatch between calf strength and the demands placed on the muscle. You can think of this as a supply–demand relationship, with not enough supply to cope with the demand placed on the muscle. Strengthening the calves can remedy this mismatch and help the Achilles tendon to heal. Doing the simple two-up, one-down heel raise exercise (*see page 248*) each day will help to strengthen the calf muscles.

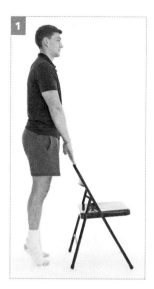 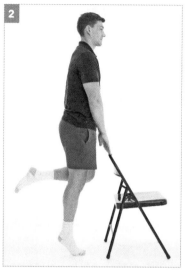 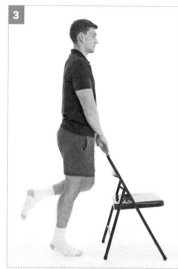

Stand on both feet while supporting yourself against a worktop or the back of a chair. Using both sets of toes, push up and raise your heels off the floor (1). Then take all your weight onto just the injured side (2) and use only that set of toes to lower your heel slowly (to the count of four seconds) back to the floor (3). At the bottom of the movement, put both feet back on the ground and repeat 10 to 15 times, several times a day.

Continue to Walk, But Don't Push the Distance

A lot of people choose to take the "no pain, no gain" approach when it comes to aches and pains. Unfortunately, more often than not, this isn't the right way forward and lands you in a worse situation than when you started. If the pain is continuing after the first 15 minutes of your walk, don't simply try to push through the Achilles tendon discomfort. Either slow down a bit or stop and rest. Try to pick a distance and pace that you can consistently walk at without setting off the pain and to stick to it.

Use Ice on the Painful Area to Reduce Soreness

Using ice over the sore spot on the Achilles tendon can improve your symptoms and help to settle inflammation. It won't "fix" the problem, but you'll certainly feel better afterward. As with all ice advice in this book, protect the skin and only apply for 15 minutes at a time.

Fix Flat Feet and Improve Your Walking

It's likely that you've heard of the term "flat feet." Maybe someone—perhaps a physiotherapist or podiatrist—even told you that you've got flat feet. But what does this funny term mean and why is it significant?

"Flat feet" (also called "over-pronation" or "collapsed arches") refers to a problem with your foot posture when standing or walking. A normal foot posture consists of the front of the foot, the outside of the sole, and the heel making contact with the ground as you stand still. A foot with good posture has an arch that doesn't make contact with the ground, which should look almost like a cave on the inside of your foot when you're standing. The term "flat feet" refers to the *loss* of that arch. This means that the inside of the foot now also makes contact with the ground, as well as the forefoot, outer sole and heel.

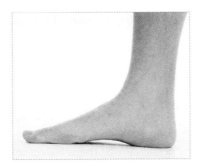
Normal foot posture

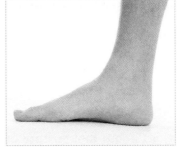
Flat foot posture

At this point, it is important to note that there is no "perfect" foot posture and there are plenty of normal individual differences.[4] You only need to consider how footprints in the sand can differ from person to person. However, with a footprint within a "normal" range, we shouldn't be able to see the outline of the entire bottom of the foot in the sand. You would see the heel, then a slim print of the outside of the sole, then the forefoot and toes. In someone with flat feet, you might see the entire foot making contact with the sand, which would make the footprints "fatter" in the middle.

But why should we care about flat feet?

As previously mentioned, our feet are like the tires on a car. They are the one area of the body that makes contact with the ground when we walk. If that contact is altered, it can affect every other aspect of our walking gait.

When you lose the arch in your foot it becomes "flat," altering the way force travels through your foot and up your leg when you walk. This means the foot, ankle, knee and hip joints all have to compensate and adapt to this change in your mechanics.

Usually, the body is clever and can adapt to these changes effectively, so much so that we often don't even notice. However, sometimes these adaptations can lead to problems. An accumulation of the suboptimal forces traveling up the leg due to flat feet can cause stress and even accelerate arthritis in our ankles, knees, hips and lower backs as a result.[5] This means that when someone finally realizes there's a problem, it's often too late.

Some people believe that flat feet are a permanent and unsolvable problem, determined by genetics. However, the truth is not quite as simple as that. It is true that flat feet are sometimes caused by the collapse of the ligaments that control our foot arch or genetic variations in our foot posture. If this is the cause, the only solution is to find a good pair of custom-fit orthotics. In other cases, though, flat feet begin as a result of the foot muscles becoming "lazy," often as a result of wearing shoes that are too supportive, too much of the time. This seems to be the case particularly for people who wore supportive footwear throughout their developmental years.[6] Supportive footwear allows the foot muscles to switch off, as the shoe is doing the job for them. These foot muscles (which usually hold up the arch) then lose their strength, which can lead to flat feet.[7]

I can give testament to this first-hand. When I worked in a hospital several years ago, my uniform policy allowed me to wear sneakers at work as I often had to demonstrate exercises to my patients in the gym. Before I started at work, I invested in some super-comfortable, highly cushioned sneakers that felt fantastic on my feet. When I walked, I felt like I was walking on air.

Several months passed and I went away for a long weekend on a walking holiday. I walked something like 30 miles in the three days I was away. I wore sturdy shoes suitable for walking, but they weren't the sneakers I'd been wearing to work each day.

I came back from that holiday with plantar fasciitis (characterized by a searing pain in my heel) in both feet, which lasted for about 12 weeks following that weekend. I couldn't understand how I'd developed this problem, seemingly out of the blue so suddenly. Then I looked at my feet, which have always been in good nick . . . and both my arches were as flat as a pancake.

Wearing my super-supportive sneakers all day every day had effectively given my foot muscles a free ride. They had switched off, refusing to do any work. And they clearly continued to refuse even when I took my sneakers off. So, when I went on my walking holiday, I had no foot strength to draw on and I developed this problem as a result. Lesson learned. I now only wear those sneakers for exercise, with a less supportive pair as my daily shoes.

If you've just looked down and realized your feet may be flat, my recommendation would be two-fold.

First, I'd recommend that you try not to always wear the most supportive shoes you can find. As long as you don't have pain, try walking barefoot around the house (especially on carpet) and wearing sandals outside of the house in the summer rather than sneakers. Let your feet do a bit of work for a change. It's the only way they'll get strong again.

My second recommendation would be for you to dedicate a bit of time to reconnecting with your foot muscles. Yes, this sounds like a very bizarre concept but hear me out. When our feet don't have to work as hard as they were designed to, we lose the ability to control the muscles within them. Have you ever seen someone with disabled upper limbs learn to paint using their feet with extraordinary skill and precision? Do you think they were born with this ability? Of course not. They put in the time to practice and now have incredible control over their foot muscles.

But before you pick up a paintbrush with your toes and attempt to paint the next Picasso masterpiece, let's start with something a little simpler. Try the following hollow foot exercise for several minutes each day, sitting with your foot relaxed on the floor underneath a table, at your work desk or while watching TV:

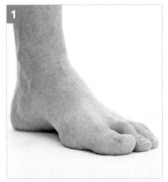 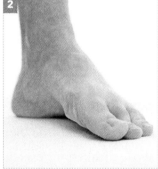

Keeping your toes and heel in contact with the floor at all times (1), use the muscles in your feet to lift your inner arch as high as you can (2). Hold for two or three seconds, then return to the relaxed position. Repeat 10 to 15 times in a row, whenever you get a quiet moment to sit.

How to Stop Twisting
Your Ankle

"I can't stop twisting this damn ankle," I exclaimed as I sat on the grass of the football training ground and held my ankle after another stomach-turning sprain. I could feel the swelling forming under my sock and knew I'd have to cut yet another session short.

Several years before I became a physiotherapist, I naively believed that I was alone in suffering the frustration of multiple ankle sprains, always on the same side. I used to put it down to being clumsy on one side; I am heavily right-handed, after all. But when I started working and saw many people with the exact same issue as me—painfully rolling the same ankle every few weeks—I finally realized I wasn't unique.

Sprained ankles become a vicious cycle for many people. You twist your ankle, the ankle becomes weak, you finally feel able to start walking on it, then you begin to exercise again . . . only to twist it again almost immediately. The cycle repeats, ad nauseam.

Does this sound familiar?

When I worked in professional football, one of our key goals was to prevent this happening to the players we looked after. For professional players, ankle sprains were commonplace, often putting them in the physiotherapy room for four to six weeks at a time. If that sprain became recurrent then it was catastrophic for the player and the team. Yes, you can strap up a sprained ankle—but if you fail to deal with it properly the first time, it has an incredibly high chance of recurrence.

So, by necessity, we developed clever ways of rehabilitating these common sprains to stop them from happening over and over again.

I often think back to being much younger and wish I had known these clever tricks when I was spraining my ankle every few weeks. I could have avoided all the missed football matches and frustration, as well as preventing the permanently stiff ankle I now suffer with, simply by putting in a little work up front. When you sprain your ankle, or any other joint in the body for that matter, you get three problems occurring all at once:

1. The Physical Injury

This refers to the damage to the ligaments (tough bands of tissue that hold your joints together) and strains to the surrounding muscles. Most ligaments and muscles heal up well over a period of several weeks, but some can heal poorly, replacing healthy tissue with scar tissue, which can lead to an unstable joint.

2. Loss of Muscle Strength

When your brain identifies damage somewhere in your body, one of the ways it protects the body from further damage is by "shutting off" the muscles around that joint temporarily. You may have experienced this after an ankle sprain; even though the bone wasn't broken, you probably struggled to put weight through your foot, as if the strength was completely gone. That is the brain's effect at work. The muscle strength does recover on its own over a few weeks—to some degree—but even when you feel strong again, there will still be weakness in certain movements or actions.[8]

3. Loss of Coordination—or "Proprioception"

The term "proprioception" means your ability to tell what position your body is in without needing to see it with your eyes. If you shut your eyes and you raise your arm up in front of you, you can tell that your arm is raised away from your side without needing to open your eyes. This is your internal proprioception system at work, and it's controlled by little receptors all over your body called proprioceptors. After you injure your ankle, your proprioceptors temporarily malfunction and fail to work as well as they did before the twist (this is one of the reasons why ankle twists can become recurrent).[8] Without proper rehabilitation, your proprioceptors will continue to function poorly, putting you at risk of further injury.

These three problems all combine to cause a problematic ankle that is prone to twisting or giving way regularly. The only way to avoid this is by encouraging the damaged ligament to heal properly and by rehabilitating the loss of strength and proprioception over a period of several weeks. The hard work is worth it if you can avoid recurrent injuries for the rest of your life (plus the risk of a more "serious" injury from a fall because of a dodgy ankle).

Here are the three steps I encourage those with an ankle injury to take to prevent consequences later down the line:

Let the Joint Heal!

Too many people, myself included, rush back into physical activity too soon following a sprain. By "physical activity," I'm referring to walking on rough terrain, exercise classes at the gym or running, among other things. All of these activities may feel all right at the time, but they represent risk. It only takes a slight slip and you're back to square one. How long you avoid these activities for is up to you and depends on how bad the initial injury was, so be sure to get advice for your own personal circumstances. You should certainly continue to try to walk and weight-bear as early as you feel able, but do this through taking short walks and pottering around at home, not by taking intense exercise.

Rebuild Muscle Strength

Of utmost importance is your effort to rebuild any lost strength around your ankle. As every sprain is slightly different, everyone has weakness in slightly different areas around their ankle, so some personalized recommendations are needed in each case.

However, the banded ankle eversion exercise below is a great strengthening exercise to help build the peroneal muscles, which are important in preventing future sprains. You can also try this exercise sitting on a chair with your legs extended in front of you.

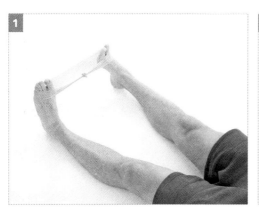 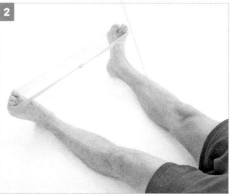

Lie on your back and stretch out your legs in front of you. Wrap a resistance band around the ends of both feet, at the base of your toes (1). Keeping your knees in a steady position, turn your feet out into the band, trying to rotate the ankle and stretch the band (2). Slowly rotate the ankles back to the start position. Repeat until you feel a working ache in your outer ankles and lower leg, several times a day.

Retrain Your Proprioceptors

As important as rebuilding your strength is rebuilding your proprioception. One important job of your proprioceptors is to allow you to balance. Therefore, any balance practice will also improve your proprioception. For rehabilitation, try the tandem stand and single-leg stand exercises on pages 203–204.

The most important thing to remember about ankle sprains is that just because the pain has gone from your ankle, it doesn't mean the problem has resolved. The injury may have healed, but you're likely to still be suffering from a loss of strength and proprioception. Early action is key, as each subsequent sprain is harder to recover from. Every sprain increases the laxity at your ankle, making future rehabilitation harder. Don't delay, start taking the right steps early and ensure ankle health for many years to come!

Reconnect with Your Feet

When we were Neanderthals, we didn't have the modern-day luxury of shoes. This meant that walking was always done barefoot. Our feet would have been toughened by hard callouses, resistant to jagged stones and hot ground.

Our feet would have been "internally" tough, too. The muscles within our feet (all 20 of them) would have been strong and well coordinated, with abundant strength to propel us forward as we walked barefoot. Unfortunately, finding someone with feet like this is a rare occurrence in today's world.

Our supportive footwear and comfortable sneakers feel great on our feet and allow us to walk and run without pain—but comfort almost always comes at a price. Over time, we have lost our ancestors' foot robustness, and the integrity of the subtle arches that enable proper foot function has suffered, too. With shoes that provide protection and support, the muscles in our feet no longer need to work as hard as they once did. Remember the old adage "if you don't use it, you lose it"? This applies to our foot muscles just as accurately as it does elsewhere.

The negative effects of a loss of foot muscle strength include increased risk of foot problems such as plantar fasciitis, greater likelihood of knee and hip problems, and possibly even an accelerated aging process throughout the lower limbs.[5,7] You're also likely to be less efficient when walking and running, if these happen to be your hobbies.

So, what can be done to counter the effects of "lazy feet" caused by modern footwear?

As noted previously, it is important not to "over-wear" comfortable and supportive footwear. Providing you don't have any pre-existing problems, it may be a good idea to make an effort to walk around the house barefoot as much as possible, or at least in flat, unsupportive slippers. Sneakers are definitely still useful, but try to reserve them just for sporting activities. Of course, this advice might need to be reversed when it comes to dealing with an existing injury, in order to give the affected area the chance to heal.

If you're someone who wears heels regularly, try to walk without them until you absolutely need to wear them. I had a client who was making an effort to avoid heels because of an ankle problem, but she had a fancy dinner party coming up the following weekend. I recommended that she wear flat shoes right up until she was about to get out of the car outside the venue, then put her heels on for the event, taking them off in the car again afterward. It worked out that she only had to walk in heels from the car to the dinner table and back, rather than all the additional walking in heels had she worn them the entire evening from her house to the event.

Another solution I regularly recommend to my clients is to begin a foot-strengthening regime. This may sound bizarre but it's actually quite simple to build into your routine. You can find my top recommended exercise for this purpose, towel scrunches, on page 159, but here's a recap: start sitting, and place the edge of a towel under your toes. Using the muscles within your feet and toes (without letting your heel lift off the floor), grip the towel repeatedly as if to pull it toward you along the floor. Once you've scrunched the towel up entirely, roll the towel back out to its original position again and repeat.

You'll notice as you perform this exercise that the natural arch on the inside of your foot has to lift to pull the towel in. This is good. It is being lifted by the muscles in your feet that may have been "switched off" for quite some time. Don't worry about the sensation of cramp as you do this exercise—it usually means you are starting to use muscles that haven't been exercised in a long time. You can find a demonstration of this exercise (plus some more ideas for improving your foot health) in Video E in the Resources section (*see page 413*).

Maintaining a good arch on the inside of your foot is an important safeguard against foot, knee and hip problems alike, and the more you practice this exercise the more permanent the change will become.

Fix Plantar Fascia Heel Pain in Three Simple Steps

As anyone who has suffered with plantar fascia heel pain can tell you, it really is a pain in the, well, foot.

As someone who has personally suffered with this problem (on both feet, no less), I can attest to the fact that it can be frustrating and even debilitating for some people.

But what is plantar fasciitis and why is it so common?

In the underside of our feet, we have a tough band of fibrous tissue called the plantar fascia that joins the front of our foot to the heel. Without this band of tissue, our feet would be shapeless, flat as a pancake, with no arch whatsoever. The plantar fascia is a very important part of our anatomy. If you think of a traditional longbow (the kind Robin Hood used once upon a time), the plantar fascia represents the bow string, while the bow itself is the rest of the foot. If the bow string isn't present, the bow loses its tension and shape very quickly (as well as becoming effectively useless until re-strung). This is a metaphor that I like to use when talking about the plantar fascia.

You can feel your own plantar fascia by feeling along the underside of your foot from the heel, along the tough, fibrous, rope-like band in the instep of your foot, under the arch. This is the plantar fascia and it can sometimes be quite tender to touch. The pain with this condition usually occurs right where the plantar fascia attaches to the heel. It can sometimes feel like the heel bone itself is painful. Pain can often be felt inside the arch of the foot, too. The layman's term for plantar fasciitis is "policeman's heel," so-called because this heel pain can be caused by excessive walking (as your typical police officer might have to partake in while walking the beat).

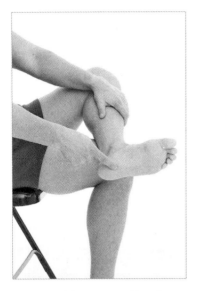

The usual location of heel pain in plantar fasciitis.

The reason the plantar fascia can become problematic for some is largely due to the mechanics within the foot. When you walk, the job of the plantar fascia is to transmit force from your forefoot to your heel as you propel yourself forward, pushing off the toes. This job is usually shared between the plantar fascia and the muscles within the foot.

Plantar fasciitis is thought of as an overuse injury and usually develops over time when we neglect other areas around the foot and ankle.

This problem can be caused by a number of underlying issues, including but not limited to:

Tightness in the Calves

Because the calf attaches to your heel via the Achilles tendon, when your calves become tight they pull upward on the heel, which makes the entire operational "unit" of your lower leg and foot (calf, plantar fascia and foot muscles) tight. This changes the mechanics within the foot.[9] Don't worry too much about the specific mechanics involved, but remember that tight calves are almost always a bad thing, especially for foot health.

Weakness in the Foot Muscles

In the previous section of this book, I talked about the reasons for foot-muscle weakness and how it can cause problems. The foot muscles share the same job as the plantar fascia. If they are not pulling their weight, the plantar fascia is subjected to more stress and strain over time.

Tightness within the Plantar Fascia Itself

While this is usually a secondary problem arising from one of the other causes, it is still an issue that needs addressing. If you feel with your fingers, as described earlier in this section, and your instep is sore to the touch, your plantar fascia is probably tight.

Poor Footwear Selection

Just to complicate matters, wearing either super-supportive *or* under-supportive footwear can directly or indirectly trigger plantar fasciitis. The key here is to change things up from time to time and never get stuck in one pair of shoes for an extended period of time.

An Injury That Causes a Collapsed Foot Arch

It is possible to injure your foot in such a way that it causes a loss of the natural arch on the inside of the foot. If this arch is lost, the way we use our feet changes dramatically and this can lead to plantar fasciitis.

Too Little Exercise, Followed by Too Much Exercise

Our bodies hate sudden changes in activity levels and they often complain to let us know about it. A sudden change in the distance, duration or pace of your walking or running can trigger plantar fasciitis.[10] This is because suddenly increasing your walking can expose underlying weakness or tightness and poor mechanics. In addition, when we push ourselves physically, our walking or running technique can often slip as we get tired. It is at this point that problems occur.

So, what can we do about an episode of plantar fasciitis? Well, the good news is that it does get better, provided you do the right things. However, although plantar fasciitis is usually self-limiting (which means it'll go away on its own eventually), if we don't address the underlying problems that caused it in the first place, we're vulnerable to recurrences later down the line.

Below are three important steps I recommend to my clients when it comes to resolving plantar fasciitis, which you can start putting into action today. Remember, with all the exercises in this section it's important to get the all-clear from your doctor or physiotherapist before putting them into action, to check they're suitable for you and your personal circumstances.

1. Self-Massage for Pain Relief

This is arguably the least important of the three steps, but I feel it can bring some value and certainly helped me when I was a sufferer. Take a hard ball, like a golf ball, place it under your foot when sitting and roll out the hard "knots" on the underside of your mid-foot and arch. This can help to relieve some of the pressure on the plantar fascia and help your foot recover faster. *Important note*: Do NOT roll over the heel bone itself with the hard ball as this will aggravate the problem.

Sitting in a chair with your foot resting on a ball, gently push down on the ball and apply pressure on the fleshy instep. You are likely to find tender, 'gristly' areas that are sore to press on. Massage these areas until they are less tender using the ball for several minutes a day.

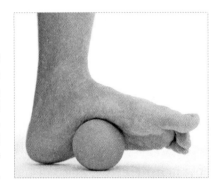

2. Stretch the Calves

Tight calves make plantar fasciitis much more likely and are probably the leading contributor to the pain. For that reason, it makes sense that stretching the calf will take some of the pressure off the foot and improve your symptoms. My favorite calf stretch can be seen on page 224. Hold the stretch for a minimum of 30 seconds, repeating several times a day.

3. Strengthen the Feet

Taking some time to strengthen the foot and the calf, over a period of time, will help your muscles to support the foot again. The exercise in "Reconnect with Your Feet" on pages 257–258 is very effective here. Another way to strengthen the feet and improve function of the plantar fascia is to attempt the plantar fascia heel raise exercise shown below, which is a variation of an exercise called the heel raise.

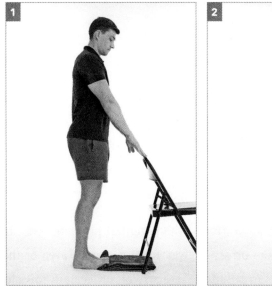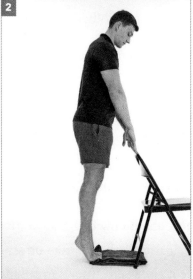

Begin by standing with your toes resting on the edge of a rolled towel. Support yourself by holding onto the back of a chair or a worktop (1). Push up through your toes and lift your heels off the ground. To the count of four seconds, lower your heels back to the ground (2). Repeat 10 to 15 times, several times a day.

By putting these three steps into action, most people can expect their plantar fasciitis to resolve within several months, or up to a year in more persistent cases. The other important thing is to be assessed and advised by a physiotherapist who can identify any weak areas and mechanical problems that you may have missed in order to prevent this condition from recurring, as it often can when not fully dealt with.

When to Use Orthotics

Orthotics are small inserts placed into your shoes with the purpose of lifting certain areas of the foot to spread, relieve or redistribute pressure. Some orthotics are firm while others are soft. You can get orthotics either off the shelf, or prescribed by a professional like a physiotherapist or podiatrist.

So, in what circumstances are orthotics suitable?

This is a more complex question than it may originally seem. At the end of this section, I've included a list of problems that orthotics have helped some of my clients with—but it's impossible to guarantee they'll work for you, too. I'd love to give you a list of injuries that orthotics always help with, but such a list unfortunately doesn't exist, mainly due to individual differences between you and your neighbor.

Let's first talk about how orthotics work and the potential problems we can run into through their use. Orthotics take pressure away from a certain area of the foot and redistribute it elsewhere. They can help to take a stretch off certain muscles, like the calves, and can almost instantly improve the symptoms of some conditions. They are useful in correcting subtle leg-length discrepancies without necessitating the use of built-up orthopedic shoes.

The problem is that reliance on orthotics for a long period of time can lead to semi-permanent changes to your movement mechanics.[11] Here's an example: imagine you feel a tightness in your calf when you walk, and you start to wear orthotics in your shoes. Upon introducing the orthotics, your symptoms disappear entirely, as you've lifted your heel and thus taken the stretch off the calf muscle. However, you've removed the symptom by effectively placing the calf into an even shorter position (you just no longer feel the tightness, as you've added some "slack" to the muscle with the orthotic) without addressing the cause. This means that, over time, your calf is going to adapt to this shortened position and become even tighter. Then, when you remove the orthotic, your problem is much worse than it was when you began.

The same story is true when it comes to fixing "flat feet" or collapsed arches: you're artificially lifting the arch with the orthotic, which helps the symptom but actually worsens the underlying problem, further collapsing your arch in the long term.

However, this isn't to say that orthotics are to be avoided; quite the contrary for many people. If a person has a genetic or structural abnormality in their foot, ankle, or even knee, an orthotic can often be a revelation in the way the person's foot interacts with the ground as they walk. This can be the difference between agony and pain-free walking for many people.

The only way to tell if an orthotic is suitable for you is to consult a professional about your own individual circumstances. In my clinic, we provide a bespoke orthotic prescription service, which will fit your feet with the right orthotic for the problem, as well as giving you advice on how to fix the problem over the long term. We always start by gaining data about how someone walks by making them take a few steps on our foot scanning machine. I have found that custom-made, 3D-printed orthotics (designed with the data we collect in the clinic) are far superior to off-the-shelf pairs.

If you're wondering whether or not to try orthotics for your problem, be sure to seek advice from someone who offers a similar service to us. Navigating the world of orthotics alone can be difficult. Shop-bought orthotics can sometimes be effective; but there is such a range to choose from that the probability of making the wrong decision is very high. Custom-made orthotics are undoubtedly better, although significantly more expensive.

Anyway, here is a list of complaints that some of our clients have found relief from by wearing orthotics as part of their treatment plan:

- Plantar fasciitis

- Achilles tendon pain

- Pain on the inside of the knee

- Lain on the side of the hip

- Bunions

- Leg-length discrepancy

- Arthritis of the ankle or big toe

- Recurrent ankle sprains

- Knee-cap pain

- Corns and callouses

- Lower-back pain

If you're currently struggling with any of these problems, get in touch with us if you're nearby (*see Resources, page 413*), or find a local expert to help you decide whether it's worth pursuing a trial of orthotics.

The Problem with Tight Calves

This is something I touched on in the previous sections of this chapter, but it is a point worth driving home again.

Tight calves are not good; they are the origin of and aggravate many problems in the feet and ankles (and even elsewhere in the body). At one of the hospitals I once worked, they offered a "calf stretch class" dedicated to treating calf tightness, delivered to a class of 20 or more patients. For such significant financial outlay to have been authorized by the powers-that-be, specialists there must have felt strongly that addressing tight calves was a priority.

The reason tight calves can be so problematic is due to the effects they have on other structures around the calf and foot. Some of the most common problems caused by tight calves are plantar fasciitis, Achilles tendon pain and pain at the back of the knee.[12] Calf pain can also be present, but—surprisingly—this often isn't a symptom. For that reason, most people with tight calves don't even realize what is causing pain in their knee, foot or ankle.

Tight calves pull at attachments on the heel bone and at the back of the knee, tugging structures away from their intended positions and stopping other muscles from doing their job. They put stress on the Achilles and the plantar fascia in the foot, leading to an exponential increase in the likelihood of problems in these areas.[13]

So, what can cause our calves to become tight?

There are probably a number of factors causing your calves to tighten up. One of them is definitely genetics, with some people being prone to calf tightness, while others don't seem to suffer at all. Another is your choice of footwear. Wearing shoes with a heel puts the calf in a shortened position—and the body quickly adapts to suit the positions we spend a lot of time in.

I also strongly believe that everyone should have a good stretch from time to time, and while most people over fifty are very good at remaining active, they are quite poor at following exercise with a good stretch afterward!

The solution to a tight-calf problem that I present to my clients at HT Physio consists of a combination of stretching and hands-on treatment. This two-pronged approach is vastly superior to just one or the other alone, in my opinion. In my estimation, combining both methods of treatment just about halves the time it takes for the typical recovery. Hands-on treatment helps to provide a rapid boost in the flexibility of the calf muscle, while the stretching done afterward helps to maintain any gain in range of movement.

If you're a walker and you wish to continue walking for many years to come, I would recommend pre-empting calf problems and addressing potential tightness long before a problem arises. I've seen people with calves so tight they were beyond conservative treatment and had to undergo a "surgical release" of the muscle to treat the problem. Avoiding surgery is always better than having to go under the knife, and early action is the key.

A great gentle stretch you can try at home to treat tight calves, provided you get the all-clear for your particular circumstances before you try it, is the calf stretch on page 224. You can also see a video where I demonstrate five different calf stretches on Video F in the Resources section.

Which Shoes Are Right for Me?

As this is something I am frequently asked about, I wanted to dedicate a short section of this book to the question of choosing the right shoes for some of the common situations we face each day. I've mentioned footwear a few times in this chapter and I understand it can be confusing when it comes to choosing the right option. Should you opt for the most comfortable? Or do you go for flat, sturdy, "sensible" shoes? This section has the answers.

However, I must preface this section by reminding you that everyone is different, so you should disregard recommendations if you have a painful problem that is aggravated by changing your shoes, or if you get contradictory advice from your own healthcare professional.

For Long Walks

I always recommend to patients that they opt for walking boots with a built-up ankle to protect against sprains and twists. Walking boots are designed to be durable and protective over long distances, so if walking is your main hobby then they are worth the investment. In general, opt for the ones that are most comfortable in the shop, as long as they support the ankle area as well as the foot. A good arch support also helps, as many people have slightly dropped arches and these can help to take stress away from the joints.

For Daily Wear

I recommend wearing a variety of shoes for day-to-day wear. Mix it up between sneakers, flat shoes and sandals—whatever you feel most comfortable in. I advise regularly changing shoes day to day, so that your feet and lower limbs don't adapt too much to any one pair of shoes, as this can become problematic. If you're in the house, on carpet, or walking in the garden on grass, feel free to walk barefoot, as long as it is comfortable. Walking barefoot is a great way to build foot muscle strength (but must be approached with caution, as too much barefoot walking can be overkill).

For Evening Wear

Taking fashion into account, I'm absolutely unopposed to people wearing whatever they like in the evenings, provided they are comfortable and a pre-existing painful problem isn't aggravated by their choice, including heels (which aren't "evil," just misunderstood!).

For the Gym or Running

Opt for sturdy running shoes with a firm sole. There are a huge variety of running shoes on the market and a lot of them have flimsy soles that you can quite easily bend and twist. Here's the rule: if you can bend the shoe in half, it's probably not protective enough for running. With sneakers, you generally get what you pay for in terms of durability and protection, but a recent study in the *British Journal of Sports Medicine* interestingly did not show a correlation between money spent and effectiveness of running shoe.[14]

One Incredible Trick to Improve Your Walking

Have you ever been worried about tripping when you walk? Have you ever felt that your legs aren't able to carry you as far as they once were? In both of these instances, there could be a simple solution to your problem.

We use many different muscles when we walk. The hip flexors swing the leg forward. The quadriceps extend the knee and prevent it from giving way. The calf muscles propel us forward. All of these muscles are important; yet there is one muscle that is almost always forgotten about but which has an equally vital role.

We call this muscle the tibialis anterior (*see below right*) and its job is to lift our ankle upward, so our toes clear the ground when our leg is swinging forward. This important muscle sits at the front of your shin and you can usually see it "pop out" when you pull your toes up toward you.

If the tibialis muscle is not working properly, tripping on the ground is more likely (as, too, are falls). A weak tibialis muscle will also lead to an increasing sense of fatigue as you walk, as if you are lacking power in your legs, with the lower leg tiring much faster than it should.

Thankfully, just like any other muscle, the tibialis can be strengthened, providing you know how. I have one excellent exercise for strengthening the tibialis, which I share with you below. I often tell my keen walker clients

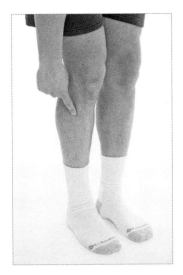

Tibialis anterior muscle

to adopt this anterior tibialis raise daily for a while. They usually report back, saying what a difference it makes to their walking. The exercise can be done up until the point of tiredness in the tibialis, which will feel like a working ache at the front of the shin.

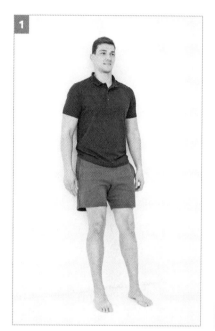 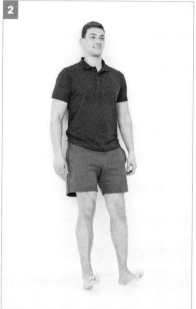

Stand with your hips and shoulders resting against a wall and your heels about 45cm (approx. 18in) away from the wall (1). Keeping your heels in contact with the floor, lift your toes on both feet up toward your shins as high as you can (2). Hold for several seconds, then slowly lower them to the ground. Repeat this 10 to 20 times, or until you feel some fatigue in your shin muscles, several times a day.

Part Seven

WHOLE-BODY HEALTH

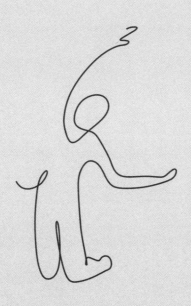

Introduction

So far, we've covered each area of your body separately in this book, giving you strategies for ensuring your joints and muscles remain healthy and injury-free. However, if I were to conclude the book here, I'd be making an enormous omission.

Our bodies aren't simply a collection of different muscles and joints that just so happen to work together. We are much more than that. We operate as one whole, complex organism, not as distinct parts. Therefore, from this point on, we're going to be thinking about our bodies as one magnificent ecosystem that thrives through a vastly complex series of chemical reactions and processes, which happen inside us every single minute.

By making small yet significant decisions about the way we live our lives, we can influence these complex processes and ensure the entire body functions as well as it possibly can. In this chapter, we're going to discuss how to limit harmful inflammation, how to improve your hormone profile (which governs the entirety of your health and wellbeing), and even how to stave off bone fragility in old age. Once we stop seeing ourselves as just the sum of our body parts and start realizing how even the smallest changes can have huge effects through a cascade of reactions, amazing things can happen.

The Problem with Inflammation (and How to Tell If You Have It)

Inflammation has become one of those common buzzwords that is almost always perceived as something negative that we should try to minimize.

Inflammation refers to a natural process in the body whereby certain chemicals are released by damaged or injured cells, causing the surrounding blood vessels to leak fluid into nearby tissues, often causing swelling. Reading that sentence, it does sound like inflammation is a bad thing; but that would be far too simplistic a view of this complex process!

Inflammation isn't always a process to be feared or avoided, and there are two main types of inflammation that we must consider before we go any further. The first type is called local inflammation. This is an inflammatory reaction restricted to the tissues in a certain area. When we exercise, for example, our muscles undergo damage, which leads to local inflammation. It is this damage, and the consequential recovery process that occurs directly afterward, which causes our muscles to grow and become stronger.

Another common situation that causes local inflammation is a sprain or strain. The first helpful step in the healing process following such an injury is inflammation.[1] The swelling that appears around a joint after you injure yourself is part of the body's plan to clear that area of debris and waste, allowing proper healing to occur. So, in many cases, inflammation isn't "bad" or something we necessarily want to avoid.

However, there are times when inflammation can be harmful to us. The second type of inflammation is called global inflammation, which describes high levels of inflammatory chemicals in the bloodstream. The problem with global inflammation is that it tends to be longer-lasting, can lead to tissue damage in many areas within the body and weight gain, and can generally make sufferers feel pretty terrible.[2] In addition to these unwanted effects, one of the main reasons I like to educate my clients on inflammation is because of the detrimental effects that global inflammation can have on healing from injury.

Some of the signs of global inflammation are multiple joint pains, puffy areas on your body (especially the face), and difficulty losing weight (or more weight gain than usual). If you have any of these symptoms, I would recommend a trip to the doctor's for a routine blood screen, which can help to identify the cause of the symptoms.

Global inflammation can be caused by several diseases or chronic conditions that are well beyond the scope of this book, but it can also be caused by our daily choices and habits. The choices we make every day impact the delicate chemical balance in our bloodstream profoundly.

As an obvious example, choosing to eat lots of sugary food for breakfast, lunch and dinner can significantly drive up global inflammation in the body and even lead to problems such as diabetes.[3] While most people know to avoid lots of sugar, there are other more-subtle choices that can also have a profound effect on inflammation.

Sticking with the diet theme, some of the "hidden" foods that have been shown to cause inflammation include certain types of vegetable and seed oils, which are often added to our foods without our awareness. Foods that are "ready-made" in stores and in many restaurants are regularly prepared with excessive amounts of these harmful oils and can promote inflammation.

Processed meats and "junk food" with high levels of trans fat have also been proven to increase inflammation.[4] I always recommend to my clients that they opt for supermarket or butcher's meat with as little processing between it being a living animal and being on your plate as possible. I'm also an advocate for free-range and organic meats where possible, but the high cost involved can often be a deterrent. A good approach can be to choose your most common meat products from the free-range and organic section. For me, opting for free-range eggs from organic chickens is a quick win, because I eat eggs every morning. I also buy my chicken free-range and organic—but the meats I eat less often, like beef, I buy in the regular range from the supermarket, simply due to cost. You may choose to purchase foods differently based on your budget, dietary preferences and ethical standpoint. The important thing is finding a healthy plan that works for you and that you can stick with.

Two other major causes of global inflammation are smoking and drinking. Most of us know about the detrimental effect to the lungs from smoking, but smoking also drives up inflammatory chemicals in the bloodstream and can dramatically slow down healing from almost any injury.[5] My advice to any smoker would be to seek an alternative, with a view to weaning yourself off tobacco and nicotine products entirely.

The other perspective to take on smoking is to analyse yourself from a behavioral point of view. Many smokers are less "chemically addicted" than they might seem, but highly behaviorally addicted.[6] This means that they associate having a cigarette with relief from a negative emotion, like stress. Getting help to change these cognitive-behavioral patterns can be a highly effective method for stopping smoking without relying on pharmacology.

Drinking heavily is also a common cause of global inflammation.[7] One of the causes of the classic beer belly seen in some heavy drinkers is actually global inflammation. Inflammatory chemicals in the blood send a trigger to the body to store fat around the midriff and our internal organs.[8] This is not a good thing—and not just because of the appearance of a large beer belly. The body type that stores fat around the middle and has that "solid" appearance in the belly is highly correlated with increased risk of heart attack and stroke.[9] While I am certainly not against a drink from time to time, if you have a regular drinking habit you'd probably benefit from cutting down. There are also resources available for people looking to cut down on drinking, including local support groups in many cases.

If you do have inflammation, the best way to relieve it is by making positive changes to your diet and lifestyle. As I'm not a dietician, the following is not a direct prescription of foods to eat or avoid, but a presentation of some of the available evidence regarding dietary changes that have been shown to help with reducing inflammation.

One of such family of foods is green leafy vegetables, like kale and broccoli. These wonderful greens can help to improve the longevity of healthy cells in the human body and can reduce inflammation, as well as provide fiber and other nutrients that are beneficial to health.[10]

We talked about vegetable oils often being a poor choice earlier, but did you know that coconut and olive oil have been shown to have the opposite effect on inflammation?[11, 12] Research shows that coconut and olive oil have anti-inflammatory effects, so making that change to your cooking may be advisable. However, remember these "healthy" oils are still highly calorific, and being overweight can also result in increased global inflammation.

The healthy fats in certain nuts, like walnuts, and oily fish, like mackerel and salmon, can also help to drive down inflammation.[13] The UK government health authorities recommend we include two portions of oily fish in our diet every week.[14]

Berries are another proven anti-inflammatory superfood. Blueberries and raspberries are great choices to include in breakfast and as snacks due to their antioxidant properties, helping to reduce inflammation.[15]

While these foods have all been shown to encourage a reduction in inflammation in the body, it's important to also address diet as a whole. Much like our bodies, a "healthy diet" is a sum of all its parts, as opposed to each choice taken in isolation. It's no good adding a few berries to your breakfast, then continuing to eat junk food for the rest of the day and still expecting a positive effect!

There is one thing that improves global inflammation in almost every case: exercise. Taking several brisk walks every week can improve health in many respects, and the effects it has on global inflammation are no different.[16] While resistance training (like lifting weights) has the effect of increasing local inflammation in the muscles temporarily, people who regularly weight train have been shown to generally have lower levels of global inflammation than those who do not.[17] There is a dedicated section on resistance training later in this chapter (*see page 288*).

Another part of our lives that can have a profound effect on inflammation is sleep. Those who do not get enough sleep are prone to higher levels of global inflammation and may take longer to recover from injuries, with a higher risk of becoming injured in the first place.[18] That begs the question: how much sleep is enough? The research on this important topic varies, but most experts recommend a minimum of seven hours of sleep each night, with a maximum of about nine hours.[19] It is important to note that, although older adults tend to sleep fewer hours in total, our requirements for sleep remain constant throughout our lives—so don't be tempted to think you now need less sleep than you once did![20]

In summary, to ward off inflammation as much as possible, keep active, eat well and get plenty of sleep, and inflammation should be less of a problem in your life.

Improve Your Hormones (for Over-Fifties)

Although I am neither a doctor nor a hormone specialist, many of my patients who are over fifty suffer from problems associated with changing hormones. They regularly tell me about some of the effects that fluctuating hormones have on their lives.

Some of the common problems my clients report to me include high cholesterol (which can put you at risk of heart disease), inflammation, weight gain, urinary leakage, loss of sexual desire, and even memory problems, all of which can often be linked to fluctuations in hormones as we age.

If you're suffering with hormonal symptoms, such as the ones listed above, the first thing to realize is this: you're definitely not alone! These problems are extremely common, and while that doesn't make them any more pleasant to deal with, it can provide some comfort to know that you aren't the only one going through this. In fact, out of 100 people, 50 will suffer from the effects of imbalanced hormones at least for a temporary period of their lives.[21]

Diet and Lifestyle

While our reproductive hormones do change naturally as we age (called menopause in women and informally andropause in men), it is also true that unwanted fluctuations in our hormones can be as a result of our lifestyle choices. For example, high cholesterol and inflammation can wreak havoc with our hormones—and both of these unwanted features can be brought about by a lifestyle of processed, sugary foods and sedentary habits. Both inflammation and cholesterol can be reduced greatly through committing to regular exercise and a diet low in sugar.[3] This would contribute to cutting away belly fat, which is our enemy when it comes to unpleasant hormonal changes. The fat stored around our middles produces inflammatory chemicals, which can negatively affect our hormones and bring about many of the symptoms associated with menopause.[22] Eating plenty of fruit, vegetables, nuts and fish can help to cut cholesterol and limit inflammation, thus helping to break down the belly fat that does so much harm.

Another lifestyle factor that has a significant impact on our hormone levels is sleep. Sleep is one of the foundations of hormonal health. Without sleep, it is almost impossible to have hormones that remain in normal levels. Consistently poor sleep is one of the easiest paths to hormone imbalance; in a recent study, it was shown that lack of sleep increased cortisol (a stress hormone), increased ghrelin (which promotes hunger), and decreased leptin (which promotes satiety).[23] There is plenty more on sleep in a later chapter of the book (*see page 300*).

The Pelvic Floor

Many women suffer from urinary leakage after menopause. Although extremely common, the women who have mentioned this often say that it can cause a lot of embarrassment. It's upsetting to hear about the loss of confidence that many people suffer because of this issue, so I wanted to make everyone aware that there is often a solution to this problem.

The muscles that control the flow of urine from the bladder are collectively called the "pelvic floor" and, like any other muscle group, this can become weak and unable to cope with the demands of its job. Luckily, as we've discussed many times already, muscles can be effectively strengthened—and the pelvic floor is no different. Research supports this fact, too. A recent systematic review on the topic found that pelvic floor strengthening exercises were 17 times more effective in treating urinary incontinence than no treatment.[24]

The exercises needed to do this job are quite simple and can be done anywhere at any time of the day. You can perform these exercises by squeezing the muscles that you would use if you were to cut the flow of urine, midstream. It might help to imagine the area between your bottom and your genitals "rising up" toward your tummy as you contract them. I would recommend alternating between fast contractions (repeated 10 to 20 times) and long, slow, holding contractions (repeated three to five times) of these muscles, several times a day, done over a period of a few months.

Low Testosterone

One of the most common hormonal problems for men as we age is a loss of testosterone. Research has shown that men's testosterone levels decline by about 1 percent every year after the age of forty.[25] Low testosterone levels have been linked to loss of sexual desire, erectile dysfunction, muscle loss (called sarcopenia), and even depression.[26]

All of these symptoms should be investigated with a blood test. However, it is important to know there are a few common causes for low testosterone that can easily be addressed. For a start, low vitamin D levels have been associated with decreased testosterone. Luckily, research has shown that vitamin D supplementation may help to normalize testosterone again.[27] Some experts even recommend that nearly everyone should start taking a vitamin D supplement. This recommendation becomes more important for those over fifty (and people who live in colder climates), due to the fact that our skin becomes less efficient at absorbing vitamin D from the sunlight as we age, so we must strive to get it from other sources.[28]

On the topic of vitamin D, there is research to show that being deficient can seriously increase your risk of dementia. In a University of Exeter study, adults aged sixty-five or older who were moderately deficient in vitamin D had a 53 percent higher risk of developing dementia; for the severely deficient, the risk rose to 125 percent.[29]

Another contributor to a loss of testosterone in aging men is a lack of physical exercise, especially resistance training. The benefits of resistance training are too great to ignore, which is why there is a section of this book dedicated solely to resistance training for over-fifties (and a free gift for you in the Resources section at the back of this book!). One of these benefits is a significant increase in serum testosterone levels following a period of weight training, as seen in a study in the *Journal of Applied Physiology*.[30]

Exercising against resistance—which I'd argue is one of the best things you can do for your body—can help to cut fat, improve strength and balance your hormones, as well as maintain mobility.[31] I usually recommend that people try to include compound exercises in their regime as much as possible. Compound movements involve more than one joint and muscle group working at the same time. Squatting, picking something up from the floor or standing up from a chair are great examples of compound movements that strengthen more than one area of the body.

Contrary to common belief, testosterone is not just a hormone necessary for male health; females need it too. Without healthy testosterone levels, women can be low in mood and struggle to maintain muscle mass. For this reason, resistance training is equally important for women suffering from hormonal fluctuations, and can stave off osteoporosis (or thinning of the bones), most common in post-menopausal women (more on that in the next chapter).[32]

Overall, it's important to remember that you aren't helpless in the face of the changes occurring in your body as you age, and there are practical solutions available to combat the effects of aging. You've got a lot of living to do yet, so let's make sure those years are happy, healthy and fulfilling.

Combatting Osteoporosis

Often confused with osteoarthritis, osteoporosis is actually a different condition entirely. Osteoporosis occurs when the bones in the body have lost mineral density and become thinner, leading to structural weakness and leaving the victim vulnerable to fractures. The main contributing causes of osteoporosis include hormonal fluctuations (especially in menopause), poor nutrition and a lack of physical exercise.[33] Notice how at least two of these three factors are within our control to some extent, which technically makes osteoporosis an avoidable disease in many cases.

Unfortunately, osteoporosis is a very common problem for people over the age of fifty and has a tendency to affect women more than men.[34] The reason women are more frequently affected is thought to be due to menopause. The depletion of oestrogen during menopause has been directly linked to loss of bone mass, which ultimately leads to osteoporosis if left untreated.[35]

Osteoporosis literally means "porous bones," which describes the appearance of affected bones when closely examined. There are certain areas that tend to be affected more than others; these include the spine, hip and shoulder.[34] As a result, these areas can easily be injured following even mild trauma after the start of osteoporosis, often leading to significant and long-lasting disability. Avoiding this condition should be of paramount importance for anyone who wants to preserve a long, active life.

So, what can we do to ward off osteoporosis as we get older?

Bone scans, often called DEXA scans, are effective at detecting bone thinning and can diagnose osteoporosis (or osteopenia—the earlier stage of osteoporosis). A good initial step is to get your bone density tested if you have any concerns, just to know where you stand currently. If you know your starting point, it's easier to make a plan. I recommend that every female over the age of fifty asks for one of these scans. Your doctor may send you for a DEXA scan as part of the follow-up process after a fracture, to check you haven't developed osteoporosis. However, this discovery often happens too late in the day to be able to prevent an injury. It's best to know early and prevent the fracture in the first place.

There are medications available for people who have developed osteoporosis, which correct deficiencies in certain minerals and help to strengthen the bones again. Nevertheless, prevention is always better than cure and if you can do it naturally, even better.

One way to ensure you are protected against osteoporosis is to make sure your diet is working in your favor. The body uses calcium and vitamin D as "building blocks" for bone, so ensuring that you include plenty of calcium and vitamin D in your diet is very important.[36] You can get calcium from dairy sources and meat, and vitamin D can be derived from sunlight as well as eggs and oily fish. If you lead a vegetarian or vegan lifestyle, you will have to take extra care to ensure you're getting enough of these vital nutrients and a supplement may be beneficial.

A "forgotten" mineral that is equally important in combatting osteoporosis is magnesium. Magnesium helps to further strengthen the bones by contributing to a scaffolding-like structure, the precursor to new bone during the regeneration process.[37] In the Western world, many of us are deficient in magnesium as our typical diets do not contain enough of this precious mineral.[38] You can increase your magnesium intake through a diet that includes nuts and green leafy veg (which also contains calcium). An alternative for those who remain deficient is to look at a magnesium supplement, although there are several different types of magnesium, with each selectively targeting a different bodily tissue.

Another mineral that is of importance to bone health is vitamin K, which helps to shuttle vitamin D to the bones where it can work its magic.[39] Recently, many vitamin D supplements have started to include vitamin K as standard, due to the important supporting effects that it provides.

Besides your diet, an incredibly important factor in keeping bone loss at bay is physical exercise. While walking and remaining generally active are good for this purpose to an extent, there is one type of exercise that trumps them all when it comes to keeping the bones strong and healthy. This type of exercise is resistance training.

Resistance training is the process of pushing or pulling against some kind of external resistance, which might include weights, your body weight, or resistance bands. We've long known about the positive effects of resistance training on the muscles, but it wasn't until relatively recently that more attention has been given to the effects of resistance training on the bones. It has been proven that our bones strengthen as a direct response to resistance training.[32] This type of exercise increases bone mass and can directly prevent osteoporosis. It's our body's way of saying, "If we're going to be lifting these weights from now on, we're going to need a good, strong foundation to be able to do so!"

For the purposes of increasing bone mass, compound exercises are again superior to "single joint" exercises. As mentioned, most of the actions you perform each day (like climbing the stairs or getting up from a chair) are compound movements, involving movement of multiple joints in your body. In the gym, compound movements include the squat, deadlift, and bench press. These exercises have been shown to strengthen the bones more than single-joint movements.

To get an idea of which exercises I consider the best and often recommend to my over-fifty clients for optimal bone and muscle health (without needing access to a gym), you can download my guide to "The Top 5 Exercises for Over-50s Who Want to Remain Strong, Mobile & Active," which is a free downloadable bonus for readers of this book. You can find a link to this free guide in the Resources section at the end of this book.

Resistance Training Over Fifty

The previous chapter brings us nicely on to one of the most important sections of this book. In this chapter, I'm going to tell you more about what I consider to be the most important type of exercise for over-fifties.

Resistance training is the process of pushing or pulling against an external resistance, including dumbbells, body weight, or resistance bands. The goal of resistance training is to safely "break down" a muscle on a temporary basis—so that when it recovers, it is stronger (and possibly larger) than it was previously. We do this by working a target muscle group to fatigue through choosing safe exercises that necessitate hard work from the muscle but put minimal strain on the joints.

Muscles are one of the most adaptable tissues in the human body. They respond to the demands placed upon them. If you were to take two months of bed rest, your muscles would respond by shrinking in size and strength, with the body making the assumption they are no longer needed. Conversely, if you work your muscles hard over a consistent basis, the body recognizes the new demands and increases the size and strength of your muscles as a result.

There are thousands of different exercises and movements to choose from when it comes to resistance training—but you don't need very many to get a good result. You can strengthen almost any part of your body with some form of resistance training and, as a general rule, the stronger you are, the healthier you are.[40] I cannot think of a single instance where having stronger muscles would be detrimental. Resistance training doesn't have to take much of your time to be effective; as little as 10 to 15 minutes daily can have a noticeable effect and is one of the principles I've relied upon to change the lives of many clients in my business.

Long gone are the days when resistance training was considered the realm of body builders and professional athletes. In fact, when asked by an older gentleman whether or not he was too old to start lifting weights, Arnold Schwarzenegger, arguably the greatest professional bodybuilder of all time, allegedly replied with, "No. You are too old *not* to start lifting weights!"

And he is absolutely right. The benefits of resistance training are too numerous to be overlooked by anyone who wants to remain active, mobile and as comfortable as possible throughout their advancing years. I should also mention that resistance training can genuinely add not just years but *quality* years to your life.

Don't just take my word for it. Here are some of the proven positive effects of resistance training for over-fifties (referenced with scientific studies to support each claim) so you can decide for yourself:

- The improvements in muscle strength seen after resistance training seem to significantly reduce the risk of pretty much any injury.[41]

- Far from making us stiff, resistance training has been shown to improve joint and muscle flexibility and mobility.[42]

- You'll lose body fat, but you'll also find it easier to keep the fat off as you will gain muscle. Having more muscle on your body raises your metabolism—meaning you burn more calories at rest than someone who is the same age but doesn't have the same muscle mass.[43]

- There is some evidence to suggest that resistance training slows down cognitive decline in older adults.[44]

- Resistance training leads to improvements in stamina, meaning you won't get so tired when out walking with friends.[45]

- Back pain can often be improved through resistance training.[46] Increased strength leads to better support for the lower back and less pain as a result.

- Those who resistance train seem to have a lower risk of anxiety and other mental health problems.[47]

- Resistance training is a great way to protect against and treat arthritis, in many different areas of the body.[47]

- Strength training leads to improvements in mobility and balance, making falls less likely.[41]

- Those who take part in resistance training generally look healthier (my opinion), and it has been proven that it helps us maintain a younger-looking posture.[48]

- Those who lift weights have a lower risk of osteoporosis—as the body lays down bone to cope with the demands of resistance training.[42]

- You'll get the wonderful side effects of improved confidence, self-esteem and body image after resistance training, which may translate to improved libido and happiness.[47]

- Your sleep should improve, meaning you can get off to sleep faster and with fewer disturbances through the night.[47]

- You'll find that daily tasks become a breeze; no more heavy breathing when you get to the top of the stairs![48]

- Resistance training has been shown to have positive effects on your heart and lungs—similar to those of cardiovascular training—meaning if you're going to prioritize one form of training, it should ideally be resistance work.[48]

Such overwhelming evidence for taking up or continuing resistance training shouldn't be ignored. I'd encourage almost everyone reading this to get started, provided they are healthy enough to do so and there's no medical reason why not. Of course, always get the all-clear from your doctor before starting any new regime.

So, how do you actually go about starting a resistance training regime?

You don't necessarily need to join a gym, although that would be a good idea if you've got one nearby. The benefits of joining a gym include access to safe, ready-to-use equipment and guidance from the staff should you need it. Being in a "workout environment" is also helpful for providing motivation. However, you can just as easily start resistance training from the comfort of your own home with minimal equipment.

For readers of this book, I've created a valuable report entitled "The Top 5 Exercises for Over-50s Who Want to Remain Strong, Mobile & Active," which I've made available as a free gift for you to download, as a thank you for reading this book. It'll give you the five best resistance exercises for over-fifties, and everything you need to keep you strong, mobile and healthy. All of these exercises can be done at home with only minimal equipment. These exercises will give you the most "bang for your buck," offering you the greatest strength and health benefits in the shortest time possible.

As a reader of this book, you can download it for free by visiting the link in the Resources section (*see page 413*).

I have also included some tips below to help people over fifty get the most out of a new habit of resistance training:

Prioritize Compound Movements

Compound movements involve a number of different muscles and joints all working together at the same time. Compound movements have been proven to build more muscle and strength, while burning more calories compared to isolation movements. An isolation movement only uses one muscle group and joint, with an example being the bicep curl. If you wanted to work your biceps, you are better off choosing an exercise like a dumbbell row, which also works all the muscles in your back as well as the bicep.

Eat Plenty of Protein

Protein provides the building blocks for new muscle mass. Without adequate protein intake, you won't gain muscle. The research is mixed on the "optimum" amount of protein to consume, but most people should shoot for at least 1g per kilo (approx. 0.2oz per pound) of body weight per day if their goal is to maintain muscle mass. To gain muscle mass, the research suggests it may be beneficial for older adults to increase protein intake as high as *twice* this amount for optimal results.[49]

Split Your Workouts into Reps and Sets

A repetition or rep is one repeat of a certain exercise. A set is a number of repetitions performed in a row, usually to the point of fatigue. You can split your workouts into reps and sets, aiming for at least three sets of each exercise, performing six to 20 reps in each set. The higher the resistance, the lower the reps. For example, if I am doing a bench press exercise, I might be able to lift about 60kg (approx. 130lb) for 15 reps, but if I increase the weight to about 80kg (approx. 175lb), I might only be able to do eight reps. The sets look different but the outcome is the same.

Progress Over Time

Progressive overload is a core principle of resistance training and relates to making your workouts harder over time to encourage your body to keep adapting. If you chose the same workouts every week, you'd initially improve but then quickly plateau. It is important to keep pushing yourself as you get stronger in order to continue improving.

Work to the Point of Fatigue

Resistance training is only effective when you push yourself. You must "feel" the muscle working by the end of the set, or adaptations won't occur. Understand that the body does not want to change—it only does so when we give it no choice but to change.

I always tell clients to keep going with a set until they feel a working ache in the target muscle. This is a good indicator that you are working to fatigue.

Short Daily Workouts or Less-Frequent Longer Workouts?

The research shows that it doesn't really matter how you split your workouts. Some people like to do a short daily workout, while others prefer to do three longer sessions each week. What matters is the total volume; that is, how much work you do across a whole week. Split your workouts up whichever way helps you remain consistent and committed.

Overcoming a Broken Bone

Unfortunately, fractured bones can be life-changing, creating temporary or permanent disability. It isn't just the physical effect of a fracture that can be so devastating but the emotional repercussions, too. If you've ever experienced a fracture, you'll know how much of an ordeal it can be. From the initial trauma, to the hospital waiting room, to the scans and X-rays, to the stiffness and discomfort, even to the seemingly heartless physiotherapist asking you to move that painful joint a week or two afterward.

However, if you've recently suffered a break, there are some important principles to know that, when applied, will give you the best chance of recovery without ongoing problems.

In general, broken bones need a period of no movement, called immobilization. What this period of time does is to allow the bone to "re-set" to its original position. To enable this to happen, the body will start to lay down new bone over the area of the break. Just as a builder might erect scaffolding before laying down new bricks on a damaged house, the body operates in much the same way. The body starts by laying down "soft" bone, which is fragile and tender. This new bone behaves like scaffolding during the healing process and needs a certain period of time to harden up into "mature" bone.

It's important to say the circumstances around every broken bone are different. An orthopedic consultant should decide on the best management plan for each person's individual circumstances. Some fractures need as long as eight weeks of no movement, while others can harden up after two weeks.

After a period of no movement, it's then imperative to start moving the injured area again when safe to do so. Movement sends a signal to the body that says we do indeed still need strong bones in that area. If you were to fracture a leg and then not move it for a whole year, the body would interpret that as a signal saying "we don't need strong bones there anymore" and would, as a result, give up on properly healing the fracture, as well as taking away density of the surrounding bone. Neither of these effects would do us much good.

This is why you might meet a heartless physiotherapist who tells you to move your affected limb even when you really don't want to! Although it probably doesn't feel like it very much at the time, it's certainly in your best interests.

Another important thing to understand is that starting to bear weight through a broken bone (after the initial "rest" period) is another way of telling the body that it needs to accelerate the healing process. This is especially true when it comes to lower limb fractures, such as a broken ankle.

If someone with an ankle fracture were to avoid putting weight on the ankle even when safe to do so, while another person with an identical injury chose to gently walk on that leg once safe, the person who made the effort to walk on the injured ankle would get back to normal far sooner. The body is an adaptation machine; it will respond to anything we throw at it. By using the injured bone, the body will make every effort it can to heal.

Now that we've covered the basics, is there anything else we can do to encourage a broken bone to heal faster?

Dietary changes have been shown to accelerate fracture healing, such as consuming plenty of calcium and vitamin D. Dairy and red meat will help with your calcium intake, and if you're vegan, look to green leafy vegetables, nuts and soy. The body creates vitamin D following exposure to sunlight, so, even though you may be injured, try to get yourself out the house if you can. Consider a vitamin D supplement if you are deficient in this vital nutrient.

An important factor that will help you return to the things you love as soon as possible is the maintenance of unaffected joints and muscles around the broken bone. I could tell you many stories about patients who have fallen and broken their shoulder, but when they first came to see me it was actually their elbow or neck that was giving them more bother. This tends to be very common with breaks in the upper limbs, as you'll often be put in a sling and told to "not move it" for a month or two. While that's all well and good for the broken bone trying to heal, the other parts of the arm also get immobilized, becoming incredibly stiff and painful as a result.

The only way to counteract this is to first be aware that stiffness will rapidly set in if you don't move these other healthy joints. That's why, in my example given about a broken shoulder, it's very important to still try to move the fingers, wrist and elbow each day in order to keep these healthy areas mobile and minimize loss of muscle mass and strength.

The same is true of fractures in the lower limbs. I've seen many patients losing almost all of their thigh muscles after a broken ankle, simply because they are unable to walk and haven't used their thigh muscles in weeks. When I was working in professional football, if one of our players broke a bone, our primary job in the early stages was to minimize muscle loss in other areas of the body while the injured bone healed. That often meant two or three hours in the gym each day, working on the muscles above and below the injured area. By doing this, when the cast came off, we were only dealing with one problem area, rather than three or four. This helped players get back on the pitch faster after the injury, a great result for the player (and the manager). I am not suggesting you need to commit hours to training each day after a broken bone, but 10 minutes here and there go a long way.

Unfortunately, in my experience many people over fifty can find themselves left to their own devices for several weeks following a broken bone, before getting only a couple of physiotherapy sessions on the NHS. While they are given just enough treatment to move or walk again, there are often still huge deficits in their strength, mobility and even independence compared to how they were before the injury. It's important not to just "accept" that things can never be the same following a fracture, especially if you haven't had thorough, in-depth treatment.

At my clinic, we often help people improve far beyond what they considered possible after being discharged from the hospital system; so, if you're not satisfied with your results, I'd certainly recommend seeking a second opinion.

The Truth about Glucosamine

Chances are you know someone who is currently taking glucosamine for joint pain. Widely available from pharmacies and health-food stores, glucosamine supplements have really exploded in popularity over the last decade. But what is all the fuss about?

Glucosamine is a natural substance found in your cartilage, which helps to make up the layers of cushioning between your joints. We lose glucosamine in the joints as we age through the process of arthritis.

It was hypothesized that taking glucosamine as a supplement would help to regenerate the cartilage within joints affected by arthritis, reducing joint pain as a result. The theory sounds great; by consuming this substance in our diets, perhaps we can replace what we've lost?

Unfortunately, it turns out that this theory has never been conclusively backed up by science. There have been numerous studies done on the effects of glucosamine on joint pain from arthritis, and the results have been inconsistent, to say the least. The largest study done on glucosamine supplementation for hip and knee pain showed no significant improvement in the symptoms of participants over a period of six months.[50] Due to the results of this study, at the time of writing, in the UK NHS workers are not supposed to recommend glucosamine formally to patients for joint health.

However, there have been different studies showing small improvements in symptoms of hip and knee arthritis after glucosamine supplementation.[51] Why the results of these studies differ is unclear. Some researchers have hypothesized that the type and dose of the supplement may be the key difference, while others have concluded the differences have been down to sheer luck and individual factors.

Either way, it's important to note that glucosamine supplementation (or any other supplementation for that matter) isn't without its risks. Glucosamine may interfere with warfarin; so, if you're taking a blood thinner you may want to reconsider self-medicating with glucosamine. Glucosamine may also affect the way the body reacts to sugar, which can have implications for those with diabetes. The research also suggests that pregnant and breastfeeding women should probably avoid glucosamine (due to the lack of sufficient evidence around its safety during these sensitive times).

Anecdotally, I have heard from some clients who feel they have benefitted greatly from glucosamine supplementation—but for every one who has told me it worked for them, there is someone else who noticed no effect at all. If you're considering starting to supplement with glucosamine, it's advisable to talk to your doctor before you begin.

Unfortunately, there is no magic pill for arthritis and the jury remains out when it comes to glucosamine. However, there are other things you can do to help, as outlined in this book. Getting a targeted exercise regime to strengthen and mobilize the painful areas can significantly improve symptoms, as can making good lifestyle choices whenever possible. The important thing to remember is that it's always worth exploring options for what can be done for your painful problem. Oftentimes, help is available if you look for it.

The Science of Sleep

Do you remember when you were younger and were quite happy to stay up all night, knowing that you could sleep until the middle of the day? For most people, entering working life puts an end to that desire to stay up late, as early mornings become a necessity. You learn pretty quickly that when you get very little sleep, you function poorly the next day.

But why, on a scientific level, is sleep so important? Do we really need eight hours each night? And what happens to our health if we repeatedly allow our bodies less sleep than we need?

To answer these questions, I turned to information from prominent neuroscientist and sleep expert Matthew Walker, who wrote a revealing book called *Why We Sleep*.[52] Walker has concluded from his research at the University of Berkeley, California, that anything less than seven hours of sleep constitutes sleep deprivation. And with sleep deprivation comes an increased risk of a plethora of health problems, including Alzheimer's disease, cancer, diabetes, obesity and poor mental health.

Walker also points out how badly we have eroded the amount of sleep we get in modern-day society. In 1942, 92 percent of the population managed over six hours of sleep per night, while only half reported getting this much sleep a night in 2017. The problem with this fact is that after just one night of fewer than five hours' sleep, the number of key immune cells (the ones that fight cancer) in our blood drops by up to 70 percent. This leaves us wide open to serious medical problems. Walker also squashes the myth that older adults need less sleep, explaining that getting sufficient sleep is an important factor in staving off the onset of dementia in many cases.

His work provides us with one of the most fascinating explanations for how sleep replenishes us that I've ever come across. In a related podcast, Walker explained how a substance called adenosine builds up in the brain during our waking hours.[53] A high concentration of adenosine building up in the brain's receptors causes tiredness. Walker calls this "sleep pressure." When we sleep, it's like "releasing the valve" and letting this pressure hiss away as the brain clears adenosine from its receptors.

Unfortunately, many people suffer from sleep problems or poor "sleep hygiene," meaning they not only having trouble falling asleep but also wake up tired. If this sounds like you, there are certainly some steps you can take to improve your sleep without needing to reach for sleeping pills.

For a start, most experts recommend that we set aside some time in the evening to wind down before bed, usually between 30 minutes and an hour (but possibly longer). During this time, lights should be dimmed, electronics (including the TV) should be switched off and voices in your household should be muted as much as possible. The effects from blue light emitted by phones and televisions have been well documented; they delay the process of falling asleep, as well as preventing deep sleep.[54]

Be sure to turn off all lights in your room before sleep, including the tiny lights emitted from electronics. Even the smallest light in your room has the potential to disturb depth of sleep. That includes the numbers on your alarm clock, the standby light on the TV, and even the blinking light on an alarm system. One of the greatest investments I made a year or so ago was to purchase a set of blackout blinds for my room, which cancel out the light from the street lamp outside my bedroom window. I almost immediately noticed an improvement in my sleep. I also sleep with an eye mask, which has also improved the depth of my sleep as monitored by my sleep-tracking device.

It has been documented that the best sleep occurs when your body temperature has dropped by about 1°C (1.8°F) relative to that of waking.[55] This means it is important to keep a cool room at night. Surprisingly, having a hot bath before bed may help with this. This is because although the hot bath causes core temperature to rise, it is the drop in temperature after you get out that seems to make us tired.

In terms of bedroom temperature, research shows that keeping your bedroom cool (below 20°C, 68°F) is the optimum temperature for sleep.[56]

Limiting caffeine after midday is also a strategy that Walker recommends. He chooses to go for such an early coffee curfew because of the long half-life that caffeine has—which is around six hours. This means that, in a healthy adult, it takes around six hours for the body to clear half of the caffeine that we've ingested. This means that even a late-morning coffee may still be active in your bloodstream by the time it comes to winding down for bed 10 or more hours later.

There are also several supplements that have been shown to have a positive effect on sleep. Tryptophan is one such supplement. Tryptophan is an amino acid found in our diets, used for the production of both serotonin and melatonin, two important hormones for healthy sleep. In a systematic review, researchers found that tryptophan supplementation helped to reduce the amount of time that a person is awake in the night after falling asleep.[57]

Although taking melatonin supplements for improving sleep has become commonplace in the United States, prominent neuroscientist Andrew Huberman reminds us to exercise caution. As the typical dosage of melatonin supplements far exceeds the amount the body naturally produces, there are concerns about the unwanted side effects that this massive dose of an important hormone can have over the long term.[58]

Another factor in improving sleep is your general diet. First, meal timings are important, with meals too close to bedtime significantly disrupting sleep quality.[59] Also, type of food matters. Diets with plenty of carbohydrates have been shown to improve sleep.[60] This might have something to do with the body's ability to use carbohydrate in the production of serotonin. If you are struggling with sleep, a very low-carbohydrate diet might not be advisable.

From my own point of view and experience, I've found that people who get sufficient sleep tend to recover from injury faster than those who report disturbed or inconsistent sleep. The reverse is also true, and many of the patients I help with chronic conditions tend to be very poor sleepers. This is backed up by research, with studies showing that sleep deprivation significantly impacts healing from injury.[61]

Based on this and the ever-growing body of research from scientists like Walker, I would certainly recommend prioritizing sleep (along with diet and exercise) if living a long, healthy life is your goal.

The Importance of
a Healthy Weight

In 10,000 B.C.E., when the earliest humans walked the earth, food was scarce. Our ancestors would hunt for food—oftentimes coming home empty-handed—and when they made a kill, every precious morsel would be eaten or put to use in some way. Food was sacred, valuable and required our ancestors to put their lives in danger each time they ventured out to look for it.

Fast forward all these millennia and our circumstances have changed quite a bit. Food is now readily available without the need to hunt, trap or kill. However, our physiology is very similar to that of our ancestors' in 10,000 B.C.E. While our environment has changed significantly, evolution has yet to catch up. This means our bodies still respond to food in the same way our ancestors' bodies did.

Our ancestors learned to identify the most valuable types of food (in terms of the usable energy it contained) by the way it tasted. Anything that contained sugar was of great value: sugar provided energy to hunt and find more food. Anything that contained fat was also highly valuable. Fat provided energy for many days and, if stored on the body, produced warmth for the winter. This is the reason why fatty and sugary foods taste so good to us now. It mostly comes down to evolution. We evolved to seek these foods and now find them very palatable, simply because sweet fruits and fatty meat were what sustained our ancestors.

This puts us in quite a difficult position in the modern day. Sugary and fatty foods are all too readily available. While availability of these once-coveted foods has changed, our physiology has not. We still crave these foods and our body still sees them as precious, which is why it can be so hard to say "no" to that slice of chocolate cake, even after a satisfying dinner.

The second problem is that, as a population, we are now the most sedentary we have ever been. We move only a fraction of the amount our ancestors would have done each day. We no longer need to hunt for our meals; we just hop in the car and drive to the shop (or order in online). This means that many of us burn significantly fewer calories each day than we consume, which leads to something called a calorie surplus, leading to weight gain.

In the UK, the general public are hammered by messages from the media and doctors that we, as a nation, should lose weight. However, unless you know the reason behind why you should heed this advice, it's easy to carry on as you are. In this section of the book, I want to make a case for why a healthy weight is important for your longevity and your quality of life. In the next section, we'll also talk about how to lose weight—even when exercise isn't an option.

So, why should we try to maintain a healthy weight throughout our lives?

Being overweight carries significant risks. As well as putting you at risk of developing high blood pressure and high cholesterol (a risky combination for heart disease), those who are overweight are more likely to develop type 2 diabetes.[62-64] Certain types of cancer also occur more frequently in those who are overweight, and we see a higher incidence of stroke in the same population.[65, 66]

Painful problems are also made worse, more often than not, by being overweight. Each extra pound you carry means an extra pound of weight traveling through any load-bearing joints, which is bad news for problems like arthritis and has been shown to lead to worse pain compared to those of a healthy weight.[67] This is just simple physics.

People who are overweight tend to have worse blood chemistry as well, meaning their injuries recover more slowly.[68] From my experience, it is often more difficult to get people better when they're overweight, compared to their slimmer peers.

But that's enough doom and gloom about being overweight! Let's instead talk about the positives of being at a healthy weight.

Energy Levels

Being at a healthy weight will cause your energy levels to rise, making you ready to tackle whatever the day throws at you. Being overweight often leads to lethargy, and diets packed with sugar can lead to a big crash in the middle of the day.

Self-Confidence

Let's face it, no one enjoys being overweight. One of the reasons for this is the self-confidence issues that extra weight can cause. Maintaining a healthy weight leads to improved self-esteem (and often a better sex life as a result).

Ease of Movement

Those who were previously overweight and are now at a healthy weight often report to me how different it is for them when they walk any significant distance or climb stairs. They remark how easy it has become since shedding the pounds, and how little their knees now creak or ache during these activities. Do you have to lose all the excess weight to get these benefits? No—most of my clients report noticeable changes after as little as 2kg (5lb) of weight loss.

Improved Stamina

Similar to the point above, it can be embarrassing and frustrating to be out of breath after climbing a flight of stairs, or to be unable to keep up with your partner when out walking. By losing unnecessary pounds, you'll have less weight on your body to carry when you walk, as well as improved heart and lung health. This means you can go on for longer before having to stop to catch your breath.

Less Risk of Injury

People who are overweight tend to have a higher risk of elevated blood sugar levels.[69] Most people know about the link between high blood sugar and diabetes, but an uncontrolled blood sugar level also leads to harmful inflammation throughout the body. This can cause injury healing to slow down, as well as making the occurrence of certain "overuse" injuries more likely in the first place.[70]

Living Longer (and Remaining Independent and Active)

A study carried out by researchers from three Canadian universities showed that obese men have a life expectancy eight years below the average, and may lose as many as 20 years of "healthspan"—that is, how long they can enjoy their life feeling in good health.[71] Staying active and maintaining a healthy weight means there's every chance you'll get to spend more quality years with your loved ones.

So, now we've made a case for why maintaining a healthy weight is vital for over-fifties, let's discuss how you can get to that healthy weight . . . even when you're unable to exercise because of time constraints or a painful problem.

How to Lose Weight—Even When You Can't Exercise

Many of my clients come to me with a frustrating conundrum: they have a painful condition. Because of the painful condition, they find it difficult to exercise. Because they can't exercise like they used to, they end up gaining weight against their will. As they become heavier with each passing week, the extra weight puts further stress on the injured area . . . making their painful problem worse. In this way, spiralling weight gain after an injury can quickly become a vicious cycle.

I'll be completely honest: losing weight when you can't exercise can be very difficult. To make matters worse, there is evidence that shows the human metabolism does indeed slow down past fifty years of age, meaning one burns fewer calories each day when doing the same things.[72] However, with discipline and persistence, it is possible to lose weight without exercise. In this challenge, knowledge is power.

When you can't take part in your regular form of exercise because it has become painful, it is first important to experiment with other forms of exercise before writing it off entirely. For example, if you find it painful to walk, try swimming. If you can't swim, try riding a bike. If you have a gym membership, try the elliptical trainer rather than the treadmill. Success will come down to trial and error, so be persistent and imaginative. To give you an example, when I had a client who suffered a broken ankle, she could no longer go to her Zumba class, which was her usual weekly exercise. Instead, we substituted the exercise from the class with a little routine she could do in a chair while holding some light dumbbells; sounds easy, but after 10 minutes, she was more than a little breathless. As soon as she was able to bear weight slightly on the ankle, we got her in the pool so she could walk up and down and swim, which turned out to be an excellent alternative.

If you really cannot exercise after an injury, the only way to lose weight is by making changes to your diet.

The food we eat is largely composed of three "macronutrients" called protein, carbohydrates and fat:

- *Protein* is made up of amino acids, which are the building blocks of muscle. Protein is very important to a number of bodily functions and is found abundantly in meat, fish, eggs and nuts.

- *Carbohydrates* provide an important energy source for us, with the body breaking down carbohydrates into glucose, which is either burned as fuel or stored as glycogen. Good sources of carbohydrate include bread, pasta, rice and potatoes.

- *Fat* is arguably the most important of the macronutrients, contributing to protection of our organs, the creation of hormones and energy production. Fat is the most "calorie-dense" macronutrient, which is why it has an undeserved reputation as something to avoid. Interestingly, you cannot survive without protein or fat for very long, but many people choose not to include carbohydrates in their diet and get along just fine.[73]

Another important factor to consider is the way we measure the energy contained within our food. We call this unit of energy measurement a "calorie." You may have noticed calories displayed on food packets. It's important to know a little about calories and what they mean to us when trying to lose weight.

Our bodies burn calories to survive. Even if we were to stay in bed all day and not move an inch, just by being alive we'd still burn a surprising number of calories simply to keep the heart and brain working. The number of calories burned increases in direct proportion to the amount of movement and exercise we do each day.

To confuse matters, even if we all did exactly the same amount of exercise in a 24-hour period, each of us would burn a different number of calories. This makes it difficult to make an estimate of exactly how many calories you burn doing a given task. The UK national guidelines state that men burn an average of 2,500 calories each day, while women burn an average of 2,000 calories each day.[74] However, this figure can vary massively from person to person. One person may see weight gain from eating 2,000 calories a day, while another may see significant weight loss from eating the same number of calories. There are many factors that influence individual differences in metabolic function. Take me (a 31-year-old male) versus my father (a sixty-year-old male), as an example. My dad is of slight build, runs regularly and is older than me. All of these factors lead to a slower metabolism at rest. I am taller, younger and lift weights as a hobby, all of which contribute to a faster metabolism at rest. Therefore, if we both ate the same number of calories—with exactly the same macronutrient breakdown—on a given week, he might gain weight while I might lose weight.

Simplistically, weight gain and weight loss simply comes down to how many calories you consume and how many calories your body burns.[75] If you consume more calories than you burn, you'll gain weight. If you consume fewer calories than you burn, you'll lose weight. However, this in isolation is too simplistic a view to take on diet. Not all meals are created equal, even if they have the same number of calories. A large plate of chicken, quinoa salad and vegetables might have the same number of calories as a fast-food meal, yet the effects on the body would be wildly different. Therefore, we need to go a little deeper than calories alone to discuss how to lose weight in a healthy way.

Let's return to the macronutrients. The macronutrients make up the bulk of our meals, but each one has a different density of calories per gram. These calorific concentrations are as follows:

- *Protein*: 4 calories per gram
- *Carbohydrates*: 4 calories per gram
- *Fat*: 9 calories per gram

Due to their high caloric content, foods containing fat were once thought of as "unhealthy." This point of view has thankfully been revised. There are several different types of fat, including saturated, polyunsaturated and monounsaturated fat, all of which are vital for the human body in sensible quantities. We should try to include foods containing these types of fat in our diets, with sources including oily fish, nuts, avocados and (preferably organic) dairy.

The one type of fat we should try to minimize is trans fat, which is found in large concentrations in certain processed and "fast" foods. Trans fats raise cholesterol and have been shown to increase the risk of heart disease.[76] Unlike the other kinds of fat, there is very little nutritional benefit to eating trans fats. Avoiding deep-fried foods, margarine and freezer pizzas is a good start.

In an earlier edition of this book, I wrote about the benefits of calorie counting when it comes to weight loss. However, recent evidence shows that calorie counting may not be as effective as first thought for weight loss.[77] A study showed that those who counted calories did lose weight from their diet . . . but most quickly regained that lost weight after they stopped counting the calories.[78] As a result of evidence like this and lived experience, I have changed my stance somewhat.

I still recommend manipulating the macronutrients that make up your diet. As a general rule, for most people it makes sense to keep protein reasonably high (shooting for something in the region of at least 1g per kg, or 0.2oz per pound, of body weight). The reason we want to keep protein intake high is because of the role protein has in building and preserving muscle mass. Keeping protein intake high will encourage the body to burn fat, as opposed to breaking down muscle mass. This is one of the reasons why crash diets are so dangerous. Yes, they lead to weight loss—but much of that lost weight is muscle mass. Keeping protein high is your best chance of preventing that from happening.

The next step is to increase the amount of fruit and vegetables in your diet. Doing this achieves a couple of things: first, fruit and veg contains micronutrients that keep us healthy. Second, fruit and vegetables contain fiber, a crucial nutrient that aids in healthy digestion and also contributes to satiety; that is, a feeling of fullness. They also help to control spikes in blood sugar.[79] This will take the edge off a rampant appetite and lead to fewer cravings over the course of a given day.

After that, one of the most effective methods of losing weight in a sustainable way is to eliminate ultra-processed foods from the diet. Ultra-processed foods include fried foods, confectionery, cakes, processed meats, mass-produced bread, some cereals and fizzy drinks. These foods tend to be energy-dense but lacking in micronutrients. They tend to be rapidly digestible and highly palatable, meaning they are moreish, but won't keep you full for very long. A diet high in ultra-processed foods tends to also be a high-calorie diet, and has been linked to obesity and heart disease.[80, 81]

Simply eliminating ultra-processed foods will often automatically reduce one's calorie intake. Whole foods make us feel fuller for longer and tend not to lead to dramatic blood sugar "spikes," which cause cravings and hunger. You might also find you feel better generally, as ultra-processed foods contribute to lethargy, middle-of-the-day crashes and digestive issues. We should aim to get our primary energy sources from whole foods such as oats, quinoa, nuts, sweet potato, brown rice, vegetables and fruit.[82]

In my eyes, the suggestions above are the simplest way to lose weight sustainably while remaining healthy. The regular "fad" diets tend to have major flaws; for example, the "weight loss tea" craze fell apart when it was shown that followers were becoming severely dehydrated. The no-carbohydrate diet was great for rapid weight loss . . . but often led to rapid weight gain as soon as the person started eating carbohydrates again. Every day there is a new "proven," supposedly superior diet released by a "specialist," but going back to basics is consistently the best method.

It's not up for debate whether weight is important when it comes to a painful problem. Stress on the joints almost always leads to worsening pain, and the effects of being obese on the body as a whole do tend to slow down healing. If you're struggling with your weight and truly cannot exercise, do go and speak to your doctor or a registered dietician to get some advice specific to your individual circumstances.

The last thing to say on this topic is to try not to become frustrated! Weight loss isn't always easy and can be a difficult process. It's quite common to see a few pounds of weight loss over the course of a few weeks, only for it to seem like you've put it all back on over one ill-disciplined weekend. Be persistent: remember, a modest loss of weight can translate to significant improvements in health and injury recovery, as well as safeguarding you from future problems.

Coffee or Tea?
Three Proven Benefits of Each

Are you a coffee or a tea person?

Coffee and tea have been a ritualistic tradition in the UK over the last several centuries. Tea was introduced to England in the 1660s by King Charles II and was predominantly a drink for the upper classes of society. By the 18th century, it was a drink for all social classes. In the UK, we have earned our reputation as tea fanatics; tea consumption is estimated to be around 1.9kg (4lb) per person, per year! However, while we are the ones with the reputation, we may have discovered tea relatively late in comparison to other areas of the globe. There are archives suggesting that the Chinese have been drinking tea since the 3rd century B.C.E.

On the other hand, it would seem that coffee was discovered by chance in Yemen in around 800 C.E. A holy man was exiled from the kingdom of Mecca, and attempted to sustain his exhausted body by eating some berries from an unidentified plant during his wanderings. The berries tasted bitter, so he roasted them in an attempt to make them sweeter. To the disappointment of the man, the berries hardened after roasting, so he tried to soften them by boiling them in water. The water turned into a fragrant, dark liquid; he decided to drink it. The story goes that he was revitalized to such an extent that he was able to continue his journey without needing to pause for rest or food for a further two days.

Coffee was introduced to England in the same century as tea, according to reports. The first "coffee house" in England was opened in Cornhill, London, and drinking coffee quickly became a ritual among middle-class citizens while discussing politics and other worldly matters.

Fast-forward 400 years, and not much has changed! We still use coffee to provide ourselves with energy and we still drink tea with friends and family. Before we had the technology to investigate the health benefits of tea and coffee, our predecessors believed there were some medicinal effects associated with these drinks. And they just may have been right.

There are proven benefits of drinking both tea and coffee, and I've picked out three of the best for each to present to you here.

Benefits of Tea

1. Tea Contains Antioxidants

Tea contains high levels of antioxidants, substances found in many foods that remove free radicals and limit cell damage within the body, protecting from "nasties" like heart disease and cancer.[83] Results of a recent study also showed that black tea had the potential to control blood sugar levels and stave off diabetes.[84] Just be sure not to undo that effect with two teaspoons of the sweet stuff.

2. Tea Can Help to Reduce Cholesterol

Tea has been shown to have potential in the battle against high blood cholesterol. A simplified view of cholesterol that many people take is that we should be trying to limit low-density lipoprotein (or "LDL") cholesterol in order to reduce the risk of certain heart diseases. In a study from 2008, researchers saw a 12 percent decrease in obese patients' LDL cholesterol just from three months of black tea consumption (without any other changes to their diet).[85]

3. Tea May Reduce Your Risk of Stroke

One study followed almost 75,000 people for over 10 years, correlating their black tea consumption with incidence of stroke. They found those who drank four or more cups of tea each day had a 32 percent decrease in their risk of stroke![86] While correlations don't necessarily point to cause and effect, medical professionals say that 80 percent of strokes are preventable by proper lifestyle choices, and this finding has been replicated in a similar study.[87]

Benefits of Coffee

1. Coffee May Protect Against Alzheimer's

There is strong evidence to suggest that the compounds in coffee (including caffeine) may help to break down the brain plaques that cause Alzheimer's disease. Researchers found that drinking coffee led to a significantly reduced risk of the disease, independent of any other variables.[88] Why this is the case is unclear. It doesn't seem that caffeine supplementation alone has the same benefit, so it could be a result of other antioxidants in the bitter stuff holding neuroprotective properties.[89]

2. Coffee May Protect Against MS

There is evidence to suggest that coffee-drinkers have a reduced risk of developing multiple sclerosis. The researchers found that this was a dose-dependent effect, with those drinking more coffee less likely to suffer from the disease.[90] Again, this may be because of the documented neuroprotective effects of caffeine, or due to a different compound, such as chlorogenic acid.[91]

3. Coffee Consumption Has Been Associated with Reduced Risk of Death

There are studies showing the benefits of all types of coffee on a range of health problems. A 2016 study showed that those who drink one to two cups of coffee a day (regardless of type) had a 26 percent decreased risk of developing colorectal cancer.[92] This may be because of compounds called polyphenols contained in coffee, which work as antioxidants. Melanoidins, created in the coffee-roasting process, may also help to improve colon mobility.

As a coffee-fanatic I may be biased, but I saved the best benefit until last if you aren't yet convinced that coffee is your friend.

In a study of over three million people funded by the National Cancer Institute and conducted over a 20-year period, people who drank one to three cups of coffee per day had an 18 percent decreased risk of death from *any* cause. Some of the diseases that were identified as having a decreased incidence in coffee-drinkers included cancer, heart disease, respiratory disease, kidney disease and stroke.[93] Not bad for a little roasted bean drink, eh?

Watch Your Step(s)

No doubt you'll have heard about the magic 10,000-steps-per-day goal pushed by the media, medical community and even the UK government over the last few years. The question is, though, where did this 10,000-step goal come from and why are we encouraged to aim for it? I'd also like to pose a different question to you here: is there a quicker, easier way to get the same benefits, other than walking five miles every day?

It turns out the 10,000-steps-per-day goal originated in Japan, in the 1960s. A Japanese university researcher became worried about the increasingly sedentary population in Japan. He hypothesized that asking people to raise their average steps from 3,500 per day to 10,000 per day would help them burn significantly more calories each week, thereby combatting weight gain and coronary heart disease. He created one of the earliest versions of a step counter (called a pedometer), which could be attached to the pocket and counted steps as it responded to vibrations.

The step counter was a success, along with the researcher's marketing strategy! Not only did Japan pick the ball up and run with it, other countries caught on, too; and before long, 10,000 steps per day was seen as gospel. It turns out that since then, there hasn't actually been much further scientific research in support of this number.

Researchers have compared the health benefits of walking, say, 3,500 steps against 10,000 steps, with the latter unsurprisingly being better for burning calories and staving off heart disease. However, there have been fewer studies comparing two higher step numbers, or whether a high step count is better than alternative exercise methods.[94]

The average person in England walks between 3,500 and 5,000 steps per day.[95] Increasing that average to 10,000 would lead to an extra 500 calories burned per day, so

3,500 extra per week. For most people (simplistically speaking), this equates to roughly one pound of body fat lost (providing one's diet stays the same)—meaning, if diet is a constant, increasing your steps from 3,500 to 10,000 each day should theoretically lead to roughly one pound of fat loss per week.

My concern around the 10,000 steps per day target, however, is that suddenly increasing your steps from a low count to a high count poses the risk of developing certain injuries. Rapidly changing your activity levels can lead to overuse injuries, like Achilles tendon problems or plantar fasciitis, which can firmly stop you in your tracks and make the whole exercise of trying to get fit pretty futile.

In a very small experiment covered by the BBC, Professor Rob Copeland from Sheffield Hallam University wanted to investigate whether asking people to do three brisk 10-minute walks per day would be as beneficial to health as asking people to walk the full 10,000 steps (but at a leisurely pace) each day.[96] The three walks represent about 2.4km (approx. 1.5 miles) of distance covered, as opposed to 8km (5 miles) with the 10,000 steps, and would represent significant time saved if it was as effective.

For this experiment, the participants in the three-walks group were asked to walk briskly and with purpose, rather than ambling along. When the results of the study came in, the three-walks group reported significantly less trouble sticking to the task than the 10,000 steps group. No surprises there. But when looking at the health benefits between the two groups, the three-walks group also came out on top. The researchers said the brisk walking group checked off more "moderate exercise" minutes than the 10,000 steps group, even though the latter group spent far more time in total on their feet.

This is only a very small preliminary study, but it gives us some important information about how it might be easier to stay fit and healthy than many media outlets (and even doctors) might have you believe. The key takeaway in this study, in my opinion, is how much more beneficial walking with intent is—to the point where you're out of breath – when compared to ambling along.

I know many of my clients are shocked by how few steps they really do take each day when they start to count steps through a Fitbit, app, or smartwatch. If you feel as though you've been quite active but still aren't even halfway to the 10,000 step goal when you check at the end of the day, it can be demotivating and make it difficult to see how this goal is achievable for those of us with busy lives. By substituting your 10,000 step goal with three brisk 10-minute walks each day, the goalposts are suddenly shifted to a much more manageable place. Based on my own experience, and the results from studies like this, I've changed my recommendations to many clients: if you're not currently as active as you'd like, will you change your goal?

Use the Sauna

As a regular sauna user myself, I might seem biased in suggesting the use of saunas. However, on this occasion, it looks as though the evidence is on my side. In this section, I want to highlight some of the overwhelming evidence supporting regular sauna use, for young and old alike.

A peer-reviewed study in 2012 showed the sauna has the potential to slash levels of norepinephrine (a stress hormone) in the blood of cardiovascular-disease patients.[97] This could be part of the mechanism behind the findings of a different study, which showed that three months of sauna use improved stress, fatigue and general health.[98] So, the sauna can almost certainly improve subjective wellbeing.

But it isn't just how you feel that improves with the sauna; there are physical effects, too. Six weeks of sauna use was shown to significantly decrease leg pain in those with arterial disease.[99] Sauna use also increases insulin-sensitivity; meaning your body can shuttle nutrients to muscles more efficiently, lowering blood sugar and helping to prevent diabetes.[100]

We mustn't overlook the neurological benefits of sauna use, either. Incredibly, people who used the sauna over four times per week had a 66.7 percent decrease in their risk of Alzheimer's disease and a 40 percent decrease in overall mortality across any given 20 year span.[101, 102] Just to clarify that last point: sauna use decreased the risk of death by any cause by a massive 40 percent over a 20-year period! Use of the sauna even reduced the death rate of a group of very unwell cardiovascular patients by 6 percent.[103]

Personally, I find that 15-minute sauna sessions profoundly help with my own wellbeing and recovery from exercise and the stresses and strains of daily life. In addition to the points I've made so far, it has been shown that sauna sessions positively affect pain scores for a range of conditions, [104, 105] and I have found using the sauna seems to reduce the time dramatically that it takes me personally to recover from injury.

Luckily, the negative effects of the sauna seem to be minimal for most people.[106] You must be a bit careful with the light-headedness caused by a temporary drop in blood pressure, so always consult your doctor before starting a sauna regime.

Stressed, depressed or anxious individuals have the potential to see great improvements when adopting sauna use, too. Besides the physical benefits of the sauna, spending 15 minutes in a quiet room to sit with your own thoughts is a wonderful way to unwind, reflect and even meditate.

If possible, to achieve the greatest benefits from sauna use, I would recommend using the sauna at least three times per week, if feasible and deemed appropriate by your doctor. In terms of duration, aim for 10 to 15 minutes each session. Give it four weeks and assess your stress, wellbeing and pain levels; if effective, it could be one of the most enjoyable ways to improve some of the problems you may currently be facing!

Reaching for the Anti-Inflammatories? Consider Omega-3

While painkillers do undoubtedly help some people get relief from painful problems, they also come with a whole host of problems. For a start, opioid painkillers such as codeine and morphine are highly addictive. They also put stress on the liver during their transit through the body.

Some of the most commonly prescribed medications for pain belong to a family called anti-inflammatory painkillers. These include drugs like ibuprofen, naproxen, and diclofenac. These drugs are not thought of as addictive, but they are known to cause potentially serious adverse effects, including stomach ulcers, gastric bleeding, and heart attacks. While they can be effective for pain, they should only be taken in the short term. Prolonged use can lead to a whole host of health problems.

So, hopefully we can agree that reliance on prescription drugs for pain relief is usually a bad idea. But is there a safer alternative?

First, as a quick and important note, I am not for one second suggesting that you stop taking any medication prescribed to you, or that you personally start any new supplement regime; I am merely reporting on findings in the evidence base at the time of writing, so you can form your own opinion and do your own research, too.

There is research to suggest that omega-3 fish oils containing essential fatty acids may well be as effective as traditional anti-inflammatory medication (if not more so) for back pain caused by disc bulges and degeneration, according to the journal *Surgical*

Neurology.[107] This study showed that omega-3 supplements have the potential to reduce the inflammatory response within the body, which may provide pain relief and improve recovery from some conditions.

The paper was published by two neurosurgeons who administered high doses of omega-3 fish oil supplements as an alternative to traditional anti-inflammatories for their patients who complained of back or neck pain. The researchers recommended participants in their study consumed 1,200mg of omega-3 fish oil per day. As most omega-3 supplements come in 300mg capsules, this is the equivalent of around four capsules, so quite a large dose. If you were to consider trying this at home, you'd definitely need to seek advice from your doctor beforehand.

The results were measured after an average of 75 days of supplementation and were very interesting:

- 59 percent of individuals had decided to stop taking their prescription pain medications because their symptoms had reduced so much.

- 60 percent stated their overall pain had significantly improved.

- 80 percent of people in the study said they were satisfied with the results they had seen.

- 88 percent of people in the study said they would continue to take the omega-3 fish oil supplement.

- Perhaps most importantly, no subjects reported any adverse effects as a result of the omega-3 supplement.

When you compare the results of this study to those of the usual painkiller trials, there are usually multiple adverse effects reported and less of a positive effect observed.

In my humble opinion, I think it's worth seriously considering omega-3 as one of the most important supplements for many people, not just those with a painful problem.

The reason for this is partly because of the positive effects omega-3 can bring to general health, and partly because most of us chronically fail to consume enough omega-3 as part of our normal diets.

However, before you reach for the supplements, there are some important points to consider. For a start, not all omega-3 supplements are created equal. Some are of far superior quality when compared to others, and quality matters greatly. It may even be harmful to take poor-quality omega-3 supplements over a prolonged period of time, due to the high vitamin A and potentially high mercury content. Some experts say that poor-quality omega-3 supplements with a "fishy" smell may genuinely have a high level of rancidity, too; not a pleasant thought.[108] I should also mention that it is almost always best to get as much of any particular vitamin or nutrient through whole food sources as opposed to supplements wherever you possibly can.

Here are some great ways to add more natural omega-3 into your diet:

- **Oily fish:** Not surprisingly, oily fish contain a high concentration of omega-3. Fish such as salmon, mackerel and sardines are full of omega-3, but you can still find a smaller amount in white fish, too.

- **Nuts:** Walnuts, cashew nuts and almonds all contain high levels of omega-3.

- **Green leafy vegetables:** Packed with vitamins and minerals, including omega-3, green leafy veg is an essential part of any diet.

- **Omega-3 supplements:** For most people, an omega-3 supplement is an easy and convenient way to include more of this powerful super-nutrient in your diet. The British Dietician's Association recommends looking for supplements that explicitly state "omega-3" rather than "cod liver oil."[109] They also recommend that the general population limits their vitamin A content to below 1,500ug/day and seeks out a high-quality supplement. Check the label of your supplements and consult a dietician for advice on how to maintain this guideline. My general advice would be that you usually get what you pay for: the cheap supermarket omega-3 supplements are often of very poor quality, so do your research before parting with your money. As a personal note, I seek an omega-3 supplement with a high EPA/DHA (the "active" ingredient in omega-3) concentration. EPA has been shown to help reduce harmful inflammation and DHA has been shown to improve brain function.[110, 111]

Whole-Body Cooling

We've already talked about the power of heating your body through use of a sauna, but did you know that harnessing the power of cold can have an even greater effect on pain for many people?

It has long been accepted that extremely cold temperatures (-67°C/-88.6°F), usually only achievable through a cryogenic chamber, are effective for reducing inflammation, dampening the experience of pain and even encouraging weight loss.[112–114] They are also very effective for enhancing range of motion and decreasing muscle spasm in people with lower-back pain. One study found that out of two groups of men with back pain who completed an exercise program, the group that was first given whole body cooling had fewer lower-back muscle spasms and a far greater range of spinal motion than the other group.[115]

So, how does this effect from cooling occur?

There are physical and hormonal effects on the human body that come about because of cold exposure. These can be so powerful that people have dedicated their whole lives to researching the healing effects of cold on the human body. Some even say that the reason Scandinavian people tend to be healthier than most other groups is partly because of the regular cold exposure in their lifestyle: ice-cold plunge pools are a way of life for some Scandinavian communities, although it's worth noting that this practice is most often done in combination with sauna use.

Am I saying you need to remove the peas and frozen chicken from your freezer and climb in there yourself? Not necessarily.

A 2015 study published in the *European Journal of Physical Rehabilitative Medicine* showed we might be able to achieve the same positive effects for people with pain in less-extreme temperatures.[116] The researchers in this study took a group of people with chronic lower-back pain and placed them in one of two cold chambers—one was -67°C (-88.6°F) and one was -5°C (23°F). Their results demonstrated significant pain relief in both conditions, but neither condition was superior to the other.

There are some effective ways of cooling the entire body for pain relief, with a view to repeating the results of that study. However, it's important to mention that cold exposure is not suitable for everyone and some people may find the cold can worsen muscle spasm rather than improve it. Although there is some evidence to suggest the cold can help muscle pain, if your pain is caused by muscle spasms you might want to skip the techniques I describe below until they settle down. This is because a cold shock can sometimes cause the muscles to tense up further. People with muscle spasm might want to opt for heat treatment instead. Be sure to check with your doctor before attempting either of the exercises that follow.

The first method involves exposing yourself to the cold with a quick five-minute cold blast at the end of a shower. The shower method sounds easy, but usually requires some build-up over a few weeks. To start with, try to endure 10-second cold blasts at the end of every shower for one week just before you get out. Build these quick blasts up to at least 30 seconds before you try the next technique.

In this method, take a shower at your usual temperature, for your usual duration of time. Before you get out, turn the hot water off and turn the cold water on full. Stand facing the water for two minutes so that it is hitting your chest. Next, drop your head forward so that the water is running off the top of your head. Finally, turn away from the shower, so that the cold water is first hitting your neck, then running down your back. Stand in this position for a further two minutes.

I have tested the optimal length of time that I felt it took to get positive effects with cold showers myself. You can certainly feel invigorated, energized and less achy after a 30-second cold blast, but the real benefits start at five-minute efforts.

This powerful technique might feel like a real challenge at first but when you get into the habit of enduring the quick blast each day, it becomes exhilarating. I got to a stage within about two weeks where I would look forward to the cold shock (I opted for mine post-workout). This method may suit people suffering from any kind of inflammation-related pain. It significantly helped my shoulder when I was suffering from a tear in the cartilage around the joint.

Eat This, Not That

Did you know that the food you eat plays a major role not just in your weight but also in how quickly you recover from injury? There are foods that encourage rapid healing by reducing inflammation and promoting general wellbeing. There are other foods that produce a cascade of negative effects, elevating blood sugar, grinding healing to a halt and causing inflammatory chemicals to increase in our bloodstream.

In this instance, knowledge is power. If you know which foods to avoid, you can replace them with the foods that will produce the opposite effect. Remember, each meal you eat provides a unique opportunity to take a step toward being pain-free, rather than away from it.

Some of the foods in the following list of recommended substitutions are already widely recognized as being healthy, while others may surprise you:

Instead of Fizzy Drinks Choose Water

Fizzy drinks contain sugar or huge amounts of aspartame (a sweetener considered harmful by many), so drink iced water instead with the juice of half a lime squeezed in. In order to recover fully from injury, we should ditch the fizzy drinks as sugar and aspartame have been shown to raise levels of inflammatory chemicals in the human body.[117]

Instead of Vegetable or Sunflower Oil, Choose Coconut or Extra Virgin Olive Oil

Vegetable oil (which is also found in mayonnaise and barbecue sauce) contains compounds that raise levels of inflammatory hormones and encourage the body to store fat. Coconut oil, on the other hand, has inherent antioxidant properties and some experts suggest its daily use can help to stave off illnesses caused by oxidization, including cancer.[118] In this way, it can actually be used to help weight loss, counterintuitively. Extra virgin olive oil has anti-inflammatory properties when used in moderate quantities and (in my opinion) makes food taste far better than vegetable oil.

Instead of Fried Processed Crisps, Make Your Own Homemade Vegetable Chips

As well as the fact that fried ultra-processed foods have usually been cooked in vegetable oil, they can lead to weight gain when consumed often—with excess weight often causing pressure on joints and worsening painful problems. As a substitute, try homemade kale crisps. They taste much better than they sound and involve minimal preparation. Place foil over a baking tray, then cover it with kale. Lightly drizzle the kale with extra virgin olive oil and salt and pepper. Place the tray into an oven on 180°C (356°F) and bake for 25 minutes. The kale crisps should be crunchy and packed with flavor, making an excellent potato crisp substitute, packed with anti-inflammatory properties.

Instead of Wheat and Gluten Products, Try Gluten-Free Alternatives or Sweet Potato

Gluten-based foods like bread and pasta have been linked with a whole slew of health detriments.[119] Some experts even believe we are all gluten intolerant (celiac) to a certain degree. Gluten-based foods can wreak havoc on the gastric tract, causing bloating, discomfort and lethargy. Why not replace your usual gluten-based foods with either the store-bought gluten-free version, or a creative alternative, using ingredients like cauliflower and sweet potato? Search for "cauliflower pizza base" online or "sweet potato burger buns," for example, for some great gluten replacement ideas.

Other Dietary Additions to Consider

- Tomatoes are packed with antioxidants, vitamins and minerals which all support the body throughout the natural healing process.

- In addition to kale, mentioned earlier, broccoli, collard greens and sprouts all hold similar antioxidizing properties, along with vitamins A, C and K. They help stabilize blood sugar levels by regulating spikes in insulin.

- Almonds, cashews, and Brazil nuts all contain high levels of omega-3, a well-established anti-inflammatory. These nuts also contain phytonutrients, which promote healing and will keep you fuller for longer when used as a mid-morning snack.

- Bok choy, common in Chinese dishes, boasts an impressive 70 different antioxidizing minerals.

- Blueberries contain quercetin, a natural substance that can ward off inflammation. These little berries have long been established as a superfood.

- Pineapple contains a digestive enzyme that helps to break down inflammatory cells. Do remember to consume pineapple only in small to moderate quantities, due to its high fructose content (more on that in the next section).

Avoid Fruit Juice

While the saying has always been "an apple a day keeps the doctor away," there may be a caveat to this. I fully accept that eating fruit has health benefits; oranges can improve your immunity and apples do contain important vitamins.[120] However, eating fruit is a far cry from drinking fruit juices, even when they are labeled 100 percent pure.

While all fruits contain fructose, this simple sugar is found only in moderate quantities in whole fruit. Despite the scare-mongering you might read online, eating three to five pieces of fruit per day is *not* likely to be enough to cause fructose-related problems, which include the risk of developing diabetes, increasing levels of inflammation and frequent energy crashes.

However, fruit juice, particularly from concentrate, does contain high levels of this simple sugar, which can have unwanted effects inside the body.

Substituting fruit juice with water is the ideal swap. As some people find drinking water unpleasant, adding a cordial or squash with minimal sugar or added sweetener can help satisfy those cravings for sweetness.

Anyone trying to lose weight should put this substitution into action without delay. People who are not worried about their weight or blood sugar but who have a painful condition of some sort can also often benefit. For example, if you are suffering from a tendon problem, there is some evidence to suggest that cutting back on sugars like fructose should be a priority.[121]

The Truth about Collagen Supplements

One of the things I am often asked about in the clinic is supplements for arthritis—and whether or not they happen to be effective. There is no shortage of claims made by supplement companies with clever marketing, maintaining their product "puts an end to pain" or "reverses arthritis." Sadly, these claims are usually too good to be true.

But before we write off collagen supplements as just another case of overly liberal marketing, it's worth diving into the research a little deeper.

Collagen is a natural substance found within our joints. A special type of collagen (called type II collagen) forms the building blocks of the cartilage that lines our articulating bones.[122] You might be familiar with the term "osteoarthritis," which describes the process of this cartilage wearing down within the joints. Therefore, the theory is that if we supplement with collagen, arthritic joints may regain some cartilage and we can slow down (or even reverse) arthritis as a result.

This has turned out to be a divisive suggestion. When I was studying for my MSc, I learned that collagen molecules are large in size, meaning when they are ingested via supplement form, they have a hard time passing through the natural barrier inside the gut. If these molecules are unable to pass through the gut, they have no way of reaching the joints or potentially improving the symptoms of arthritis.

When I came to the above conclusion, my research into collagen supplementation pretty much stopped there. But in 2021, I came across a systematic review study that suggested collagen supplementation significantly improved the quality of participants' skin, hair and nails in just 90 days.[123] This challenged my understanding: if the molecules were unable to pass through the gut, how could they have such an effect? I decided to look deeper into the literature about how collagen supplementation can impact the joints.

I discovered there have been some findings in recent studies to suggest that collagen supplementation may be worth a second look when it comes to easing the symptoms of arthritis.

In 2019, a systematic review study was published by García-Coronado and colleagues that concluded that collagen supplementation was effective at reducing both functional deficit and self-reported pain in sufferers of arthritis.[124] However, this finding was not consistent across all of the studies included in the review, so there may be subtle differences in certain types of people (and certain severities of arthritis) that dictate effectiveness.

In 2021, a second review study seemed to support the findings of the first.[125] Khatri and colleagues found that collagen supplementation seemed to reduce joint pain and improve mobility after injury in a mixed population comprising both athletes and older people. Could it be that collagen supplements can improve the rate at which cartilage within the joint both heals from micro-injury and regenerates after arthritis? This would possibly explain why both sufferers of arthritis and younger but injured individuals seemed to see benefits from the treatment conditions in these studies.

In the aforementioned review, Khatri and colleagues managed to compare data from studies that measured the rate of collagen synthesis after supplementation. They found that at a level of 15g (0.5 ounces) of collagen supplementation per day, the rate of collagen synthesis inside the body was elevated. This could be one of the mechanisms for action; although more research would be needed to confirm these findings.

But before you reach for the first collagen supplement you can find, there are some important points to consider. While most collagen supplements seem to have a relatively benign adverse-effects profile, collagen supplements (like all supplements) are almost always untested and unregulated. This means you are going by the word of the manufacturer when assessing quality and content. It is a well-known fact that many supplements in powder form have a high heavy metal content. Chronic use of a supplement that has been contaminated in this way may damage health. There are also some mild but common side effects of collagen supplementation, according to research by Versus Arthritis, including a feeling of heaviness in the stomach and diarrhea.

A better option might be to increase your consumption of whole foods that are naturally high in collagen. Such examples include bone broth, sardines and skin-on chicken breast.

As with all supplements, thorough research and a dedicated review from your primary care physician is recommended well before commencing any new supplement. While the research into collagen supplementation is promising, the actual mechanism of action is not yet established—so consideration is needed before adding it to any dietary regimen.

How to Gain Muscle Over Fifty

Has anyone ever told you that it is "impossible" to gain muscle over the age of fifty? If they have, they're mistaken.

In a comprehensive review of the available literature in 2004, the researchers Hunter, McCarthy and Bamman concluded that older individuals absolutely can gain muscle in response to exercise—while also underlining how vital this is for health.[126] In fact, while resistance training is often thought of as a younger person's game, it may be even more important for health in the older individual than it is for the young adult.

Gaining muscle has been associated with improved strength, vitality, overall health and even a longer life.[127] It has been correlated with reduced rates of depression and anxiety, better libido, reduced risk of falls and injury, not to mention improved confidence in one's appearance. However, there is no denying that gaining muscle does become more difficult as we get older, so knowing how to go about it is key.

As we age, both male and female testosterone levels decrease, making muscle gain (also known as hypertrophy) more difficult. Combining that with the well-documented deterioration in the quality of muscle tissue and an elevated risk of injury, the older person does undoubtedly have to plan carefully if they wish to make significant gains in muscle size and strength.

The most important driver of hypertrophy is undoubtedly resistance training. Moving your body against its own weight or an external object is the only way to send a signal to the muscles that they need to grow in order to match the demands you are placing on them. Research shows that between three and five moderate to high intensity resistance training sessions, targeting the whole body over the course of a week, seems to be the optimum dosage for muscle growth.[128] Interestingly, in the Hunter et al. study, the researchers noted that too much cardiovascular training (running and cycling, for example) might actually impede the process of muscular development in older individuals. This could be because too many calories were being burned over the course of a day to allow for muscle growth (more on that in a moment). If you wish to gain muscle, the researchers recommended capping cardiovascular training sessions to no more than three per week to avoid unwanted impediments to hypertrophy.

The second key component to gaining muscle over the age of fifty is to be in a very slight calorie surplus. A calorie surplus is a situation where you are eating more calories than you are burning each day. The amount of surplus for optimum muscle gain is usually between 300 and 500 calories per day.[129] This seems to be about the right amount of additional calories for the body to start building new muscle, without also gaining too much unwanted body fat! If you were to resistance train and eat 1,000 more calories than you burn each day, you'd build muscle . . . but you'd also gain a belly in the process. Keeping the calorie surplus only very slight is the sweet spot.

One of the biggest differences between training over and under the age of fifty is the care and attention we should give to avoiding injury. Over the age of fifty, our tendons lose some of their structural integrity, making strains and tendinopathies (problems with the tendon) more likely. I would expect an older weight-trainer to need at least twice or maybe three times the warm-up duration of a younger trainer. A warm-up routine would include a range of mobility and "priming" exercises (designed to wake up the target muscles), followed by several sets of the working exercise with very little weight, just to practice the proper mechanics of the movement. This routine might require 10 to 15 minutes at the start of each workout.

For individuals of any age looking to build muscle, getting adequate sleep is vital. Without adequate sleep, muscle hypertrophy becomes almost impossible. For most people, this means getting at least seven hours of sleep each night.

Besides resistance training, my experience is that walking regularly and maintaining an active lifestyle are key to maximizing muscle growth and "functional" strength. Being able to move big weights in the gym but not being mobile on your feet is a hollow victory. It also seems that being generally active helps to encourage muscle growth, simply through the process of using those muscles more regularly. My hunch is that someone who goes to the gym for an hour every day, but then spends the rest of the day on the sofa, would not gain as much muscle as someone who remains active throughout the day in addition to their gym routine.

It is also important to be realistic with your goals when it comes to gaining muscle. Even if you found it easy to build muscle when you were in your twenties, it is going to take a lot longer now to see results, regardless of whether your diet and training are optimized. For this reason, it is vital that you enjoy your exercise regime, not just for the purposes of seeing changes to your physique. The trainer who actually enjoys her session will outlast the trainer who hates the workout and only does it to see results in the bathroom mirror.

Top Tips for Fat Loss

Knowing how to safely and effectively lose unwanted body fat is a vital skill for people of any age, not least people over fifty. There are several reasons why we should take this topic seriously. For a start, losing unwanted body fat becomes more difficult with age, as the metabolism slows down over the course of your life. A person who could go on a sugar-loaded binge and not notice any difference in their twenties may not be able to get away with the same behavior in their seventies.

Second, it has been proven time and again that carrying excess body fat can play havoc with our health. There is, of course, the undeniable contribution of physics: carrying more "dead weight" means more pressure on the joints, often exacerbating the discomfort of arthritic problems. But it has been proven in studies that those who carry extra fat around their mid-section tend to have higher levels of inflammation in the body, causing or contributing to unwanted health problems.[130] This is not to mention the effects that carrying excess weight have on confidence and mobility. Therefore, it can only be beneficial to know how to lose unwanted body fat at any stage in life.

There are some universal rules that apply to fat loss, regardless of what is in fashion in the weight loss space. One such rule stems from the laws of thermodynamics, and states that an excess of caloric intake (eating more than one burns) will lead to weight gain, while a deficit of caloric intake (eating less than one burns) will lead to weight loss. However, fat loss is a little more complex than just eating less than you burn, as we discussed in a previous chapter. Modern research shows that while simple calorie counting does work for fat loss, it is difficult to stick to from a behavioral perspective.[131] It is also true that not all calories are created equal: if you were to eat 1,000 calories' worth of ice cream, this would have a significantly different effect on your appetite and energy levels than eating an equal number of calories comprised of "whole" foods.

There is also the argument that ultra-processed foods contribute to weight gain more than their "whole" food equivalents. Ultra-processed foods are anything that has to be significantly modified before it reaches the consumer. The issue with ultra-processed foods is that they have effectively been "predigested" by a machine, making them hyper-palatable and quickly metabolized at the same time. This effect leads to a spike in blood sugar followed by a crash, which then causes significant hunger later in the day. The cravings, of course, will draw the victim toward more processed foods, thus repeating the process.

Another more recent area of research that we should all be aware of is the gut microbiome. It has been shown that the gut contains over 1kg (2lb) of live bacteria within it at all times.[132] This community of bacteria is known as the "microbiome" and its effects on health have only recently been acknowledged. There is now evidence to show the brain and the microbiome are inseparably linked, with the microbiome actually influencing our food-seeking behaviors. It is important to understand that the microbiome changes, depending on what we put into our bodies; if we feed it sugary snacks, the bacteria in the microbiome will rely on sugar as an energy source, thus driving cravings. If we consistently feed the microbiome healthy whole foods, however, the cravings for sugary snacks will begin to disappear. In this way, it is possible to manipulate your appetite and cravings simply by changing your eating habits and waiting for the microbiome to catch up.

Although I am not making any claims to be a competent dietician, I want to share some practical tips for how over-fifties can turn the information above into a strategy for fat loss, should they choose to. Below are some of the science-backed fat loss tips I often find myself recommending to my clients:

Always Keep an Eye on Calories

Even though other factors are undoubtedly important, if you consume more calories than you burn, you will gain weight. It helps to track calories over the course of a week to give yourself a rough idea of your daily average. If you are gaining weight, you are eating more than you burn. If you are losing weight, the opposite is true.

Prioritize Resistance Training

Many people make the mistake of thinking that a calorie deficit is all that is needed to lose fat. In the absence of resistance training, you'll lose almost as much muscle as fat.[133] This is a negative, so preventing muscle loss while you lose fat is vital. The only way to do this is by sending a signal to your muscles that they are still required. You can do this through resistance training. Research shows that resistance training forces the body to spare muscle tissue and burn fat instead, while also increasing your metabolic rate. Win–win!

Prioritize Protein

This is another tip that will help you to maintain precious muscle mass while losing fat. Protein molecules are the building blocks from which muscle tissue is made. If we don't have adequate protein each day while in a calorie deficit, the body will break down muscle tissue to provide it. You can prevent this from happening by consuming enough protein each day (the ideal amount will vary from person to person).

Prioritize Whole Food Sources (and Minimize Ultra-Processed Food)

Choose foods where there are minimal steps between the food being grown and ending up on your plate. Avoid processed foods, or food with lots of unnatural additives. A wise personal trainer once said, "Only accept it on your plate if you can pick it, pluck it, or skin it." With some exceptions, it is difficult to go too far wrong with this rule.

Keep Your Steps Up

Reducing your caloric intake is only one side of the equation; the other is increasing the number that you burn each day. Walking is a great exercise for satisfying this side of the puzzle. While 10,000 steps is a common goal, there is actually little science behind this exact number. Start with a walking distance that feels achievable, then build up from there.

"Cardio" Is Not Mandatory

Contrary to common belief, running, cycling and swimming are not mandatory for those who want to lose fat. Yes, they will help you to burn more calories—but it is entirely possible to lose fat with just diet and a healthy lifestyle. One problem with lots of cardiovascular exercise is that it can change your metabolism to be more "efficient" over time, meaning your body can survive on fewer calories. This sounds like a good thing, but it can be detrimental to fat loss, as you'll need to eat less and less over time to be in a deficit. While cardiovascular exercise is a great way to build fitness, its effect on metabolism is one of the reasons I tell people to prioritize resistance training, which has the opposite effect and can actually speed up metabolism, at any age.

Find Healthy Snacks

Snacking in and of itself is not a bad thing to do; it is the composition of that snack that makes it helpful or harmful. If you know you like to snack, be sure to have some healthy options in the house for when you get peckish. Preparation is half the battle when it comes to fat loss. If you have a low-calorie snack available (such as my personal favorite, oats with Greek yoghurt), that will keep you fuller for longer, and you'll make it to the next meal time without too much worry.

Consider Intermittent Fasting (IF)

For those who struggle to lose fat, IF can be an effective strategy. IF is the process of confining your food intake to a predetermined window of time each day. For example, you might choose to eat only between the hours of 11 a.m. and 7 p.m. While the mechanism behind how IF works is still up for debate, it is a simple fact that most people end up eating less in total if they put these restrictions in place.[134] A commonly chosen window is eight hours on, 16 hours off. The window can be made tighter if faster results are desired.

Don't Deny Yourself Too Harshly

Finally, remember that you are being restrictive in order to improve your health and wellbeing, not to self-flagellate. If you fall off the wagon, don't beat yourself up; just take the next opportunity to hop back on. Equally, sometimes it is a good thing for morale to allow the odd "cheat meal" consisting of your favorite treats. As long as this isn't done too often, it shouldn't significantly hamper your progress.

How to Get Up from the Floor

Research by the King's Fund states that falls directly and indirectly cost the NHS over £2 billion every single year.[135] Falls are a huge problem in the population of patients that I treat in my clinic. They are a leading cause of injury and long-term disability for over-fifties all over the world—and, in most cases, we are woefully unprepared for them. It is not too dramatic to suggest that preventing a fall truly is a matter of life and death. It is sad but true that a third of people who fall and fracture their hip will die within the next year.[136]

So, preventing falls is vital. We have already spoken about strategies to prevent falls—such as training your balance, building strength and maximizing mobility. But despite taking preventative measures, many of us will fall at some point in our lives. That is where this section may well come in handy.

Much of the trouble associated with falls comes not from the impact of the fall but from the inability to get up from the floor after falling. It is entirely possible to prevent some of the morbidity associated with falls if we can all learn how to get up from the floor ahead of time, should we ever be unlucky enough to be down there in the first place.

Aside from falls, many of my clients report to me how they are shocked to discover that they can easily get down to the floor . . . but they were caught in a sticky situation when they were unable to get up again! This often happens when weeding the garden, or trying to get something out from under the bed. The realization that you are stuck can be frightening. The information below aims to prevent this from being the case for you, and remedy it if you have already noticed difficulty in getting up from the floor.

These movements will need to be modified in some way if you have a bad knee or hip, so they may not suit everyone. However, they are the most effective method for rising from the floor once you find yourself down there.

If you would prefer to see this sequence of movements in video form, I have two videos on my YouTube channel which demonstrate a) the movements required to get up after a fall and b) a training program that will help you develop the strength and mobility required to get up from the floor. You can find links to these important videos in Video G and Video H in the Resources section (*see page 413*).

Note: Only attempt this exercise if you have someone in the house to help you if you struggle to get up by yourself.

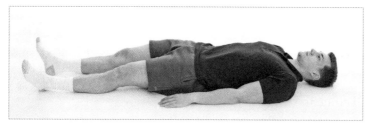

1. Start by lying on your back on the floor.

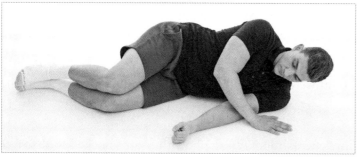

2. Bend both knees and then roll onto one side.

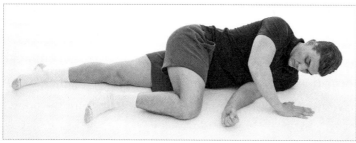

3. Bring one knee up toward you and straighten the other, rolling toward the side of the bent leg. Place your hand on the floor in front of you and your bent knee on the ground.

4. Bring one knee up toward you and then roll onto it, using the knee and your hand to lift your body from the ground.

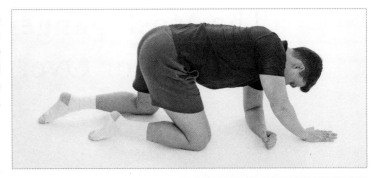

5. Continue to bring the leg through and place the foot on the floor, then rise to a kneeling position.

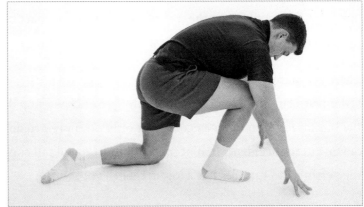

6. Push down through the planted foot and rise up to a standing position.

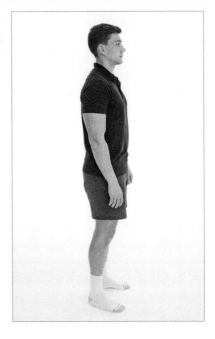

The Most Dangerous Movement for Over-Fifties

There is one particular type of movement that is responsible for more injuries than any other in people over the age of fifty, leading to particularly traumatic falls. The movement we are talking about is stepping down from a height.

There are many times throughout the day when we must step down from a height to a lower platform: situations like descending stairs, stepping down a curb or stepping off the bus all fall into this category. Not only do more accidents happen when stepping down, but the accidents that occur from this type of fall can be far worse in severity, as the person who tumbles has a lot further to go.

There is one major reason why stepping down is so dangerous, and it has to do with the demands this movement places on the body. To understand it properly, we must first understand a few principles about how our muscles contract.

There are three types of muscle contraction:

- **Concentric:** This is when the muscle shortens as it contracts (e.g. the way the thigh muscle contracts as you climb the stairs).

- **Isometric:** This is when the muscle contracts but does not change length (e.g. the contractions in your finger muscles to carry a bag of shopping).

- **Eccentric:** This is when the muscle contracts while also getting longer (e.g. the way the thigh muscle contracts as you descend a flight of stairs).

Research has shown that the third type, eccentric contractions, are the most demanding on our muscles.[137] And it is eccentric contractions that are required for any stepping down movement.

An eccentric contraction acts like the "brakes" of your body. It slows down movement against gravity. If you did not have the ability to contract a muscle eccentrically, you would be able to climb stairs . . . but when trying to come down again, you'd have no choice but to suffer the full effects of gravity every time.

It has been shown that (when we do nothing about it) we lose 3 to 8 percent of our muscle mass with each passing decade after the age of thirty, with more severe losses after age sixty.[138] One of the most critical losses to the function of our muscles is in our ability to contract them eccentrically, meaning we lose some of our ability to hit the brakes. This means we can no longer fully control our ability to safely lower ourselves down to the floor. If you have ever experienced the feeling that your knee might give way on the stairs or when coming down a curb, it could be the first sign that you are lacking in this essential eccentric strength.

Here are some other signs that you are lacking eccentric strength and are thus at risk of a nasty fall:

- Your legs feel "weak" when coming down stairs.

- You have to hold the rail when going down a step.

- You are fine climbing hills, but dread coming back down.

- You are unable to control your descent slowly onto a chair or the toilet.

- You notice your knee falls "inward" toward the midline of your body when you come down stairs, or descend into a chair.

Thankfully, even if you notice all of the above signs, all is not lost. It is absolutely possible to regain your ability to descend stairs and steps safely in a matter of a few months, with practice.

I have two favorite eccentric exercises that will help. The key to these exercises is that the downward part of the movement should be done slowly. If it is rushed, the entire object of the exercise is defeated. These exercises should be practiced little and often, ideally every day. Only do them if they do not cause pain (and make sure it is safe for your individual circumstances to do so). The first exercise, the sit-to-stand, is demonstrated on page 205. The second exercise, the eccentric step, can be seen below:

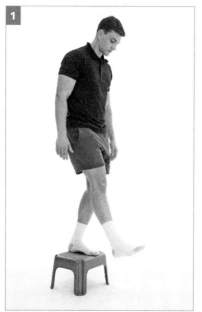
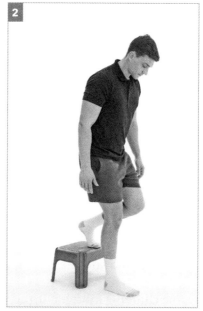

Stand on a bottom step (or a small step like the one above). You can hold on to your banister for safety if needed (1). Move your weight onto one foot and slowly lower your other foot down to the floor to the count of four seconds (2). Return to the start position and then repeat with the other leg.

12 Tips to Fix Your Walking

One sentence I find myself often remarking to my clients is: "You never expected to have to relearn to walk, did you?"

While I say it in jest, I do spend a lot of time teaching people how to walk "correctly" at my practice. And I can assure you this isn't because the people I'm coaching aren't intelligent or capable; these are educated people who have been walking their whole lives. It's because walking should be seen as a skill that one must learn, just like a golf swing or a tennis serve.

Too many of us take walking for granted. We imagine the correct way to walk is to just put one foot in front of the other. We have done it this way for years, so why should we change now? Unfortunately, this is the wrong way to approach walking. If we continue walking with subtle bad habits, there is a high chance that we are putting undue stress on our joints, activating the wrong muscles and even leaving ourselves open to a greater risk of falls. You might get from A to B—but you'll be risking a lot in the process.

Instead, it pays to learn how to walk correctly. You don't necessarily need to see a physiotherapist to fix your walking. Below are 12 "checkpoints" I look for when assessing someone's walking gait. All 12 of these steps are required for healthy, safe and pain-free walking. See how many you can check off in your own walking:

1. Heel Strike

The first thing that should strike the ground when you walk is the bottom of your heel. If you aren't touching the ground first with your heel, it makes all of the other components of walking difficult. A heel strike sets the foot up correctly to "roll" forward onto the toes, thus allowing you to push off as you take steps forward.

2. Hip Extension

Once you have your foot in contact with the ground, as your body travels over your foot, you should use your buttock muscles (glutes) to push your standing leg out behind you and propel you forward. Many over-fifties lose their ability to extend the hip, which means they must compensate by overuse of their spinal muscles, often leading to back pain.

3. Toe-Off

You should then push off your toes, using your calf muscles to drive your body forward. Many of us become "lazy" with our calf muscles, especially following an injury. This leads us to lift the foot, rather than using the toes to push. If this is the case, you lose a lot of power and walking becomes more difficult.

4. Knee Bend

When the opposite leg is traveling through the air ready for the next heel strike, one common mistake is not to bend the knee as it is airborne. This makes catching the foot on the floor more likely and a trip can occur as a result.

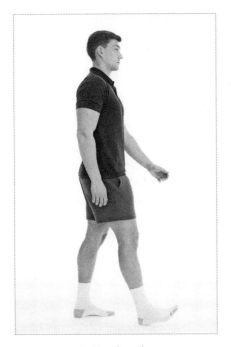

1. Heel strike

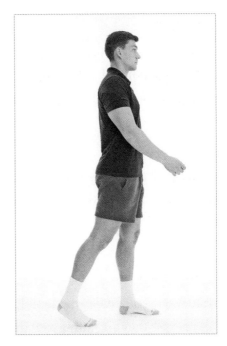

2. Hip extension

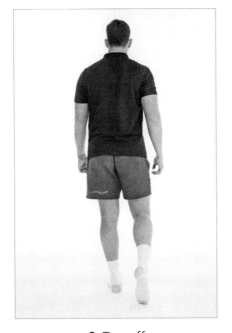

3. Toe-off

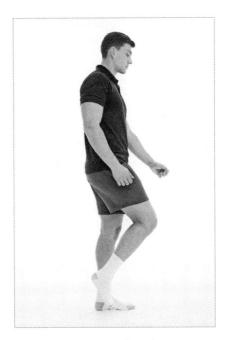

4. Knee bend

5. Stable Hips

When walking, it is important not to allow the hips to drop to one side. If this occurs, it gives the appearance of a "bottom wobble" during walking. This is a sign of weakness in the glutes and it puts a lot of stress on the side of the hip and the inside of the knee.

6. Gluteal Squeeze

As we walk (and especially when propelling forward with the trailing leg), we should feel an active squeeze in the buttock muscles which generates power and spares the lower back.

7. Tummy Tuck

Have you ever seen people who look like they have a big belly when they walk? This could be because they are failing to activate their "core" muscles, which act like a corset to keep everything in the abdomen in place. Without this core activation, an anterior pelvic tilt (which looks like a duck bottom) can occur, which tightens the hip flexors, disadvantages the glutes and stresses the back. The answer? Pull your tummy in very slightly as you walk while also focusing on activating your bottom muscles as you go.

8. Chest Out

Many patients I speak with in the clinic worry about their posture when walking. They notice that they have become more hunched when walking and don't like how this makes them look and feel older. The answer is often simple: raise your chest up and out, lifting the shoulders and head. This will instantly improve posture.

9. Arm Swing

One big mistake I see seniors make when walking is that they stop swinging their arms. Your arms act like a counterbalance when you walk, with the right arm swinging when the left leg makes contact with the ground. Without this essential counterbalance, you lose power in your walking and suffer compromised balance, too. Allow the arms to swing naturally when walking for best results.

10. Shoulders Relaxed

This will help with the point above. One of the things people often do when they try to swing their arms when walking is induce unnecessary tension in their shoulders. This will defeat the purpose of the arm swing and cause neck and shoulder pain if left unchecked. Allow the shoulders to drop away from the ears when walking, which will make your gait look and feel more relaxed.

11. Chin Tuck

Another tip to prevent neck and shoulder pain when walking is to tuck your chin in gently as you walk, as if to make a barely noticeable double chin. This is important for posture as it stacks your head perfectly on top of your shoulders. No need to draw the head all the way in; just 25 percent of the way is fine. This simple tweak improves posture, restores balance and prevents pain in the neck for many seniors when walking.

12. Eyes Gazing Ahead

Many seniors I meet have fallen into the bad habit of looking down at the floor when they walk. This is a major problem because, although it feels safer to look down at the floor, it actually makes walking more dangerous. Looking down at the floor pulls you into an unbalanced position and brings your center of mass forward, leading to a higher risk of falls. It also reduces your awareness of what is going on around you. The answer is to focus your gaze on the floor no less than 4.5m (15ft) ahead of you.

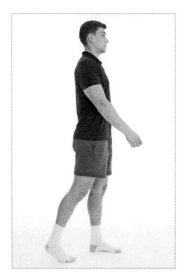

12. Gazing 4.5m (15ft) ahead

This is the sweet spot for examining the terrain ahead while also keeping a perfect posture during gait.

If you would prefer to see these steps laid out in video format, you can find a video of me walking you through these 12 steps on my YouTube channel. See the Resources section (*page 413*) and Video I.

Improve Blood Flow in the Legs

Poor circulation is a major issue for many people for a variety of reasons. Problems with the heart, lack of mobility and past injuries can all lead to compromised circulation in the legs, which can result in swelling, discomfort and reduced function in the legs and feet. In the worst instances, poor circulation in the legs can lead to a breakdown of the skin and even lead to risk of a deep vein thrombosis (DVT), which can be fatal. Thankfully, improving leg circulation is often possible, provided you know how.

It pays to first understand a little about how circulation in the legs really works. Our circulatory system works with the help of three major types of blood vessel: arteries, veins and capillaries. Arteries take blood away from the heart, delivering it to the tissues where it can provide oxygen and other vital elements. Capillaries are tiny vessels that exist near the tissues that provide the means of exchange. They have a single-cell wall, which allows oxygen and carbon dioxide to be "swapped" between the blood stream and the tissues, enabling our muscles to function. After this transfer has occurred, veins take deoxygenated blood back toward the heart. Then the process repeats.

Most people understand that the heart pumps blood through the arteries by contracting, which gives us our heartbeat. This means blood flows strongly through the arteries. However, once it reaches the capillaries, blood flow is forced to slow down in order to squeeze through these tiny channels. Once the blood has passed through the capillaries, there is reduced "pressure," meaning it is difficult for the blood to get back up to the heart through the veins. This is especially the case in the legs, where the blood also has to travel against gravity to get back to the center of the body. Thankfully, we have a built-in mechanism that stops blood from pooling in the veins in our legs, called the muscle pump. Because blood pressure alone is unable to return the blood back up to the heart, we need instead to rely on our leg muscles to help with this important job.

The muscles in the calves and the thighs act like a pump, contracting around the veins as we move our limbs, squeezing the blood toward the heart. This happens without our awareness every time we walk, stand and move. To assist us further, our veins have little "gates" built into them, which open to allow blood to flow upward but close when the blood starts to trickle back down, preventing any backward flow.

This mechanism is highly effective in improving the blood flow in our legs. However, it requires something conscious from us, too: movement of our legs. If we aren't moving our legs by contracting our muscles, the muscle pump won't work. This is why DVTs and other circulation-related issues happen more commonly in hospitals and on long flights, where people are static for prolonged periods of time. The reason these issues occur is because the muscle pump has been switched off.

So, the most important step in improving your leg circulation is to move: walking is best, but moving your feet when sitting still is also effective.

Below are a few other tips for improving your leg circulation. Share these tips with someone who has poor leg circulation, or who doesn't move as much as they should—it might just save their life:

Move Your Feet

Even when sitting down, you can keep your feet moving. By briskly bending and straightening your ankles, you activate the muscle pump in the calf muscle, which helps with blood flow in the lower leg. These movements are called ankle pumps:

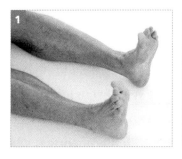 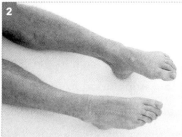

Sitting in a chair or lying on your back, briskly flex your ankles up (1) and down (2) for a couple of minutes, several times a day.

Elevate Your Ankles

Keeping your ankles elevated helps to "drain" the blood away from the ankles and uses gravity to assist with returning it to the heart. I usually recommend that clients with poor blood flow keep their feet above the level of their hip when resting.

Elevating your ankles creates the optimal position to assist blood flow in the legs.

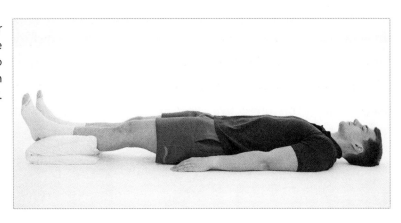

Try Seated Heel Raises

One of my favorite calf-strengthening exercises can also be used to flush blood from the calves and reduce swelling, while significantly improving circulation:

Sitting in a chair, lean forward and rest your forearms on your thighs, putting some weight through your arms. Using your toes, push down onto the floor and lift your heels up as high as you can. Slowly return to the start position, then repeat up to 20 times, several times a day.

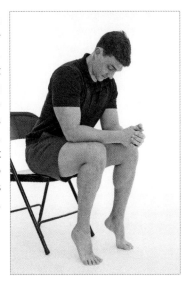

Standing Heel Raises

For those who are confidently able to stand, the plantar fascia heel raise exercise may be better. You can find this on page 263.

Compression

In some cases, compression socks are a good idea to help with circulation. These socks are similar to the kind offered on flights for the purposes of preventing DVT. They squeeze the calves and reduce the likelihood of clots during flights by almost 50 percent.[139] This protective effect also works on land for those who do not walk very much.

Part Eight

THE POWER

OF

THE MIND

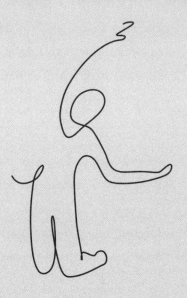

Introduction

Not too long ago, the medical profession believed that pain was always the result of physical damage. If you had pain, it was because there was a physical, tangible and measurable problem. By that logic, we also believed that the moment said injury resolved, the pain would disappear without a trace.

However, there was a problem with this theory. The advent of modern imaging technology revealed that it is entirely possible for someone to feel pain with a complete absence of any detectable physical injury. What's more, we found lots of people who had very obvious injuries that showed up on scans—but no pain whatsoever.

In the modern day, medical imaging technology has improved vastly on basic X-rays. With the advent of the MRI scan, we can now pick up on more physical problems in someone's body than ever before. This has led to the use of MRI scans as the preferred diagnostic tool for many problems.

We initially thought that, in the case of those with a painful complaint, we would be able to see exactly what was causing the problem with our clever scans, thus leading us to a clear plan for fixing it.

Except, to the befuddlement of the medical profession, there were daily exceptions to this rule. People were in pain—in the absence of any discernible injury showing on their MRI scan. To make matters more confusing still, other people had no pain—yet on their scans, we found degenerative discs, joint arthritis and even vertebral fractures!

An important study carried out by Brinjikji and colleagues in 2014 looked at the spines of a population of healthy individuals who were not complaining about any kind of back pain.[1]

The researchers took these people and performed a full spinal MRI on each. The results were astonishing.

The researchers found that, out of 3,110 people:

- Up to 96 percent of these (pain-free) subjects had disc degeneration.

- There were disc bulges in 30 percent of the 20-year-olds and 84 percent of the 80-year-olds.

- There was a disc protruding from the spine in up to 43 percent of these pain-free people.

- There was evidence of "wear and tear" in nearly everyone.

And yet, despite all the focus in pain science being placed firmly on physical problems for hundreds of years, people with seemingly horrific imaging results stood before us—without any pain whatsoever. What's more, this study is not a one-off—it has been replicated time and again, including areas of the body other than the spine.[2, 3]

So, how do we explain the reasons for some people experiencing terrible pain when they are seemingly in the exact same physical state as someone who is pain-free? There is clearly more at play than just the physical.

The human brain is a fantastic creation. It allows us to think, feel, process and understand. It can also amplify or suppress pain signals based upon past experiences, current mood, subconscious fears and vulnerabilities.[4]

This chapter is all about learning how to harness the power of the mind to control your pain. If you can use your mind to your advantage, it can work with you as a powerful ally, helping you control your pain, ease anxiety and even improve your happiness.

Some of my greatest client success stories started off with a sceptical individual resisting this approach. Too many times to count, these individuals end up becoming believers in the power of the mind by the end of our time together.

Each one of the following tips has been carefully considered. I have distilled these tips down to the ones I feel are most effective. I would recommend trying them all for at least one week (unless otherwise stated) before passing judgement. Of course, some will take longer to work than others. Some may give you an instant boost, while others will take practice and patience. Some will not be suitable for your circumstances, so as with everything in this book, seek professional advice first if you're not sure. Without delaying any longer, here are my tips for using the magnificent capabilities of your mind to help you unlock your body and ease your pain.

Your New Mantra

Of all the emotions that a human being can possibly experience in the context of pain, one of the most harmful, without doubt, is fear.

Fear, in the context of a painful problem, causes us to avoid movements and activities that are safe and necessary for a complete recovery. One of the strongest types of fear is the fear of getting physically hurt; the fear of damaging the vessel we live in.

This type of fear lies beneath the surface—we aren't necessarily aware of it—which limits our grip on the fear, even when we are determined to control it. Even if you don't feel afraid, your brain may be subconsciously avoidant of the actions that have previously caused you pain, whether it was bending forward to pick up something off the floor, using the vacuum cleaner, or walking to the shops.

Our brains are programmed to learn. We learn through experiences, with any experience that has caused us significant pain (or enjoyment) being the most influential of teachers. It is entirely reasonable to develop fear toward a movement that caused you pain in the first place. After all, your brain is designed fundamentally to protect you from danger. Developing fear, and consequent avoidance, of a situation that the brain interprets as "dangerous" is a mechanism designed to protect you.

However, there is one thing that our brains are programmed to believe that isn't necessarily true. Your brain is programmed to view anything that causes you pain as physically damaging to your body. Lorimer Moseley (an Australian world-renowned back-pain expert) explained this phenomenon using one of his personal experiences.[5]

He recounted walking through the long grasses near his home, when he felt what he assumed to be a twig on a fallen branch jab him in the calf.

Thinking nothing of it, he continued his walk.

As it turned out, the "twig" that had jabbed him was a deadly brown snake sinking its fangs into his lower leg. Lorimer ended up in hospital, fighting for his life, in desperate need of anti-venom.

Luckily, he lived to tell the tale. The next time he went walking in a grassy field, he genuinely did get jabbed by a twig disguised in the long grass. On this occasion, for a split second, he recounts feeling incredible, searing pain. Once he looked down and saw that it was, in fact, just a twig that had jabbed him, the pain instantly subsided.

Why was his reaction this time so different to his casual reaction to the genuine snake bite months earlier?

It was because Moseley's brain had adopted a learned response, etched into his mind by such a significant experience. Failing to respond to the jab in the leg the first time almost cost him his life. The second time, his nervous system would not allow the same mistake to be made.

Your brain is no different. If you've injured your body, your brain is on high alert, subconsciously looking to steer you clear from anything that represents a threat. At the first sign of this threat, your brain is going to protect you in the only way it knows how—by producing pain, which tells you to STOP! This response is evident to anyone who has suffered lower-back pain. You might find that bending forward causes a sharp jab of pain in your lower back. This pain isn't necessarily occurring because you are causing damage or even tugging at an injured area; it is simply there as a warning sign to tell you there is potential danger in this movement.

How do you stop this reaction and ease the unnecessary pain caused by your brain trying to protect you? It takes work, but there are a few methods that can help. One such method is breath timing. I have observed many of my clients (especially with back pain) tend to hold their breath when moving. This serves to increase the sensitivity of the nervous system, putting it on high alert and leading to a higher chance of it interpreting a movement as "dangerous." Instead of holding your breath while you move, if you are able to, time your breath throughout a usually painful movement; it often helps to calm the central nervous system and reduce the pain. The way to put this into action is to take a deep in-breath to the count of 5.5 seconds (claimed to be the one of most calming breathing cadences by researcher James Nestor), then breathe out to the same tempo as you start the movement.[6]

If you find the pain you feel as you move starts to make you fear movement in general, I've found a simple mantra that may help to alleviate this reaction when repeated in your head.

This mantra is designed to work on movements that you could once do without pain but are now difficult. For example, this may help someone with back pain who now fears bending forward to put their socks on, or someone with knee arthritis who fears walking due to the nagging pain on the inside of their knee.

The mantra is this:

"Pain does not equal damage."

Next time you feel yourself aching at the mere thought of carrying out an activity that you find painful, remind yourself that pain does not equal damage. For it to work, you must truly believe it. And, thankfully, for many chronic conditions, this mantra is true. Research has shown that knee arthritis, many lower-back issues and certain types of chronic neck condition can cause pain on movement without any additional injury occurring.[7] For these conditions, as long as you've been given the all-clear for your individual circumstances, movement is generally safe (and advisable), so keeping this mantra in your head might allow you to move enough to improve the condition. Just repeating a certain phrase can solidify our belief in it, so keep reinforcing it with regular repetition if you find it useful.[8]

I've found this tip to be effective for people with conditions like fibromyalgia, if used over the long term. Fibromyalgia can cause unexplained pain, seemingly with no rhyme or reason behind what hurts and what doesn't. Reminding yourself that your pain doesn't always mean you are causing physical harm should help to ease the anxiety associated with ongoing pain, as well as potentially easing the pain itself.

Learn to Meditate

What do you think of when you hear the word "meditation"? Do you think of Buddhist monks sitting cross-legged on a hard, stone floor for days on end chanting "Om"?

Fortunately, meditation for us average folk doesn't need to be such a feat of endurance, nor does it need to be spiritual if you don't want it to be. Meditation is the act of taking a short period of time to focus inward. Reassuringly, you don't need to become "enlightened" to gain some benefit from this practice. Meditation is a very simple process and the best part is, you can't meditate "wrong," because there is no "wrong"!

There are many types of meditation available to choose from, but many focus around concentrating solely on either noticing your breath entering and leaving your body, or paying attention to the sensations that arise as you sit quietly. Most people prefer to sit still in a quiet place while they do this, but there's no reason why you can't focus on your breathing while going about your daily errands. When done consistently for even 10 minutes each day, I've found there to be a tangible sense of relaxation as a reward, extending long beyond the meditation time itself.

Meditation has been used to manage pain for hundreds of years by Buddhists. The effects of meditation on pain management have been, at last, tested in the West. In a 2018 review, the authors found that mindfulness meditation reduced self-reported pain significantly in chronic pain-sufferers.[9]

The authors of the aforementioned study attributed this to a change in the way the brain processes pain, reducing the unpleasantness of the experience. No matter which way meditation works, the cost of adding meditation into your daily routine is minimal. All it takes is 10 to 20 minutes of your time and a quiet space.

Most people opt to undertake their meditation practice first thing after they wake up, as the mind tends to be clearer before the hubbub of everyday life begins. Having a meditation practice that you engage with before you check your phone, read the newspaper, or answer emails means you avoid falling into "fire-fighting mode"—the state of frantically trying to solve seemingly imminent problems—before you have had time to set your mind up for the day.

I believe that meditation must be performed consistently over a period of several weeks before you really start to feel the positive effects. Don't expect to keep your mind calm for 20 minutes without becoming distracted. The act of bringing your attention away from distraction and back to the breath is the practice. Some meditation masters suggest that achieving even one truly focused breath per day is a good start!

Try the meditation practice below for several weeks before evaluating the effects:

- Find a quiet place to sit. You can choose any position, but it is better to be upright (as you'll be less likely to fall asleep!). Close your eyes and focus on taking three deep breaths. Notice how the air enters and exits through your nose, how it rushes into your chest. Notice the area of the body that rises and falls as you breathe.

- After these three initial breaths, with each new breath focus on a different part of the body. Simply observe how this part of the body feels as you breathe in and as you breathe out. Be very specific. For example, don't just focus on your hand. Focus on the second knuckle of your third finger. Change your focus each breath.

This tip is perfect for those suffering from chronic, low-level anxiety, which has been shown to significantly exacerbate painful problems. We know that anxiety can worsen physical pain so, by putting measures in place to control it, we can have a direct effect on physical pain too.

What's more, meditation has profound effects on productivity—taking the time to get your thoughts in order first thing in the morning can set up your day to be an ordered success rather than a chaotic scramble.

There is also some solid evidence behind the positive effects of mindfulness meditation on chronic headaches—researchers at the Baqiyatallah Hospital and Headache Clinic in 2018 found that mindfulness improved levels of disability and quality of life, and reduced distress in chronic headache sufferers.[10]

For more on meditation, I highly recommend downloading a meditation app which will guide you through the process in audio format. The one I use is called *Waking Up*, created by meditation expert and neuroscientist Sam Harris. His daily meditations have helped me many times to quiet my mind and center my attention on the present.

How Stress Can Accelerate Aging

We all deal with stress every single day. It's a part of life and sometimes stress can even be a good thing; certain types of stress spur us on to take action. If you've ever found an overdue bill (threatening a hefty fine) under a stack of papers, you'll have experienced this sudden rush of stress-induced urgency. However, there is another, more insidious type of stress. The type I am talking about exists persistently, just beneath the surface. Chronic, low-level stress can be harmful in the long run to both physical and mental health.

When we think of stress, we think about someone on the verge of a mental breakdown, at risk of "snapping" at any moment. While we all occasionally experience times like this, they usually pass within a matter of hours without any undue damage to our health. Beneath the surface, low-level, continuous stress, however, is a different ball game. This type of stress often goes undetected for long periods of time. It can be driven by a family problem, like watching the sad decline of an aging family member, or at work, such as when we are put under sustained pressure with a looming deadline.

I like to think of this type of stress as water simmering in a pot on the stove. Slowly, the heat builds and you start to see bubbles, which at first burst harmlessly when they reach the surface. However, if left unchecked, the boiling water can bubble up uncontrollably and even dislodge the lid covering the saucepan. When stress reaches boiling point, it's already too late—and similar to the example above, there's often a mess to clean up afterward!

Low-level, unremitting stress can have a number of effects on our health, some of which we don't necessarily notice, or even associate with stress.[11] Stomach not feeling quite right? That's often stress-related. Did you think those headaches were down to not drinking enough water? Again, it could be stress simmering away. Have you lost your energy or sex drive? It could just be that you're getting to bed too late . . . but if there's a lot going on right now, you might need to look inward instead.

Stress causes a lot of these effects on your body by releasing a hormone into your bloodstream called cortisol. Cortisol is a "fight or flight" hormone—meaning it is designed to force us to take action. In 50,000 B.C.E., when our ancestors were chased by prehistoric beasts, cortisol made sure they could get away quickly. Unfortunately, our physiology hasn't changed very much since then; so, when someone shouts at you at work, your brain sends the same signal to the adrenal glands that your ancestors would have received when chased by a hungry predator. That leads to the release of cortisol into your bloodstream at a similar dosage to the life-threatening situation. After all, your brain has perceived a threat in exactly the same way as it would have done thousands of years ago. While you don't necessarily feel like getting up and running away, the effect on your body is the same.

Over time, this repeated dumping of cortisol into the bloodstream, day after day, month after month, can lead to permanent health problems.[12] Cortisol causes the body to switch off non-urgent systems, such as your immune and digestive systems, in favor of supplying energy to your heart and muscles. Great when we are running from danger—but not good when occurring repeatedly over long periods of time. Chronically elevated cortisol causes our immune system to reduce its function, leaving us vulnerable to infection and possibly even cancer.[13] We're also less able to extract the nutrients we need from food, as the digestive system cannot function optimally in this state. Chronic, long-term stress has also been linked to anxiety, depression, heart disease, weight gain and memory impairment.[14]

So, what can we do to "switch off" the ancient mechanism embedded deep in our brains and avoid this low-level, continuous fight-or-flight response?

Experts say the following can help:

Eat, Drink and Exercise

Eating well, staying hydrated and regular exercise can all help.[15] Successful motivational speaker Tony Robbins advocates the approach of making changes to the body first, which then encourages the mind to follow. If you've ever felt low, then gone for a brisk walk or run and not felt so bad after, you'll have experienced this at work.

Learn to Relax

Learning to relax with yoga, tai chi or meditation has been shown to significantly relieve stress in a wide-ranging population across a number of studies.[16] Most towns have plenty of choice when it comes to classes and I advise my clients to look into finding one to suit their needs. The best part is, the techniques you learn from these classes can be used outside the class whenever you need a boost.

Make Time to Play

Scheduling time for your favorite hobbies, or even just to read a book, is important for managing stress. The key word in the previous sentence is scheduling. These activities need to be planned in advance, or they simply won't happen. When I started writing this book, I decided I was going to try to write a page or so whenever I "got a moment" to do so. Guess what? It never happened. So, I started scheduling one hour every morning before work to sit down and write. I found the process relaxing and rewarding (and ended up completing the book on schedule, too!).

Interact with Others

Fostering and maintaining healthy relationships may be the most important factor in controlling stress. Research has consistently demonstrated anxiety and depression rates to be higher in lonely individuals.[17] Sharing our worries with trusted companions is important and allows us to lift the lid from our "stress saucepans," even just for a moment. But it needn't all be doom and gloom that we share in order to benefit from a friend's company. Good times are equally important and allow you to switch off from the problems you might be going through in your life right now.

Laugh It Out

Laughing and stoking the fire on your sense of humor is vital. Watch a comedy, or go and meet a friend who can always make you laugh. It's a great release valve for chronic stress when you put the world to rights with a healthy dose of humor. Ending the day with a comedy series or funny book will help to reduce your stress far more than watching a scary movie or the news before bed. How you feel when you go to bed often influences how you feel when you wake up.

Seek Support

If you feel weighed down by the stress and strain of life and can't see a way out, seek help. There are trained professionals who specialize in helping people with problems like yours. They can support you in finding a way through. If you're in need of someone to talk to, your local clinic should have information about free services in your area. If you have the means to pay for counseling, I've yet to meet anyone who has been through the process of therapy and described it as a waste of money. A skilled therapist can help you work through issues that you may not even realize are affecting you.

What Science Says about Stress and Health

Intuitively, it seems obvious that stress can be detrimental to our health. We have probably all heard of someone who carried work-related stress for too long and suffered a heart attack or a similar health event. Indeed, there are some professions that have much higher rates of adverse health events across the board.

This begs the question: is minimizing stress the only way to ensure good health throughout life?

Scientific research shows the answer is a little more complicated. Take one of the many real-life examples as an interesting data point. There are people in extremely stressful lines of work who seem to tolerate the stress far better than even those in low-stress jobs. For example, US Navy SEALs—during their infamous BUD/S training—are subjected to incredibly high levels of physical and emotional stress, yet many emerge more resilient to stress, as opposed to suffering because of it.[18] There are countless other examples of individuals and groups in high-stress professions who seem to come out the other side of high-stress environments unscathed.

This fact suggests it is not the stress itself that is harmful, but how the individual deals with that stress. The research literature also supports this finding. In an enormous analysis of over 50,000 US adults, researchers found those who held the belief that stress negatively impacted their physical and mental health had a 43 percent increased chance of mortality from any cause.[19] This astonishing finding suggests that it is not the objective level of stress that is harmful to the mind and body, but whether the individual perceives that stress to be harmful that leads to adverse health problems.

US Navy SEALs were found to have a fundamental belief instilled into them during training: that stress is a positive force for change that actively makes them better. They see stress as a powerful input that stimulates growth, physically and emotionally. Rather than seeing stress as harmful, they see it in the same way you might see a hard session in the gym: unpleasant in the moment, but beneficial to your development in the long run. Research suggests that we might therefore do well to adopt this mindset in challenging times—and hold firmly in our minds the idea that stress has the power to make us stronger and more resilient in the long run, if we let it.

Another thing research seems to suggest is that many people find positive and healthy ways to relieve pent-up stress so that it never adversely affects their health. Taking physical exercise, getting enough sleep and the use of activities like the sauna all seem to be effective at relieving the potentially negative effects of stress. It might be helpful to see stress as a type of pressure that accumulates over time, with these healthy strategies being ways of "opening the valve" and releasing some of that pressure. These two approaches—adjusting our fundamental beliefs about stress and finding healthy ways to relieve it—may be the key to protecting both our inner peace and physical health in an ever-increasingly stressful world.

Use the Incredible Power of Touch

When you've suffered from pain for longer than 12 weeks, there are certain physical changes that occur in your brain and nervous system.[20] These changes can be the reason why some people find their physical injury has healed, yet their pain continues.

These changes are characterized by heightened sensitivity in the nerves, both around the problem area and in the spinal cord. This sensitivity can cause pain to continue, even in the absence of physical damage.

Unfortunately, this can cause people to spiral into a vicious circle:

- You start to feel pain, often from an initially innocuous injury.

- This pain causes your nervous system to become hypersensitive, so the pain gets worse.

- This increase in pain causes your nervous system to become more sensitive, leading to even more pain.

- The cycle repeats, ad nauseam.

These cycles are extremely hard to break. However, one of the most powerful tools we have in our arsenal is the power of touch, especially from a loved one.

Amazingly, when loved ones spend time together, their heartbeats and breathing patterns tend to naturally synchronize.[21] The effect of being with someone close to us doesn't end there. Touch can truly be a healing power. In a 2017 study, Dr Pavel Goldstein, a postdoctoral pain researcher in the Cognitive and Affective Neuroscience

Lab at Colorado University, compared a woman's painful experiences both with and without her partner's touch. Dr Goldstein found that the touch of the woman's partner significantly reduced the magnitude of her painful experience, more so than him just being present with her but not holding hands.[21]

What caused such a profound change? The researchers felt the level of trust between the couple played a significant role. The woman experiencing the pain had enough trust in her partner to believe that he was physically sharing the pain with her—and we all know that a problem shared is a problem halved.

Interestingly, this also seems to be the case when receiving treatment from a therapist. Research shows that a patient must trust their therapist in order for hands-on treatment to be effective.[22]

By having someone we truly trust lightly touch a painful area, often with no more than the weight of a feather, the nerve signals this produces can help to calm the nervous system, reducing pain as a result. Asking a loved one to perform this simple act for you while relaxing in front of the television can make a world of difference to your symptoms.

Their touch is effectively telling your nervous system: "Be calm, everything is OK. Look, this touch is safe and comfortable. You don't need to be on edge."

Into Practice

Lie still on your side or back, either with some relaxing music on or in front of some light-hearted television.

Have your partner or trusted friend sit behind you, lightly brushing your back with their fingertips, moving slowly across your skin.

If it feels like a massage, they are pressing too hard!

Ask them to perform this for up to 30 minutes. You should feel a deep sense of relaxation which grows as time goes on. Do this daily for a week and re-evaluate your pain at the end of the week.

This technique requires patience but is primarily aimed at those suffering from what we call "central sensitization"—a painful response that may be caused by neuro-inflammation, or the response of the nervous system, rather than the injury itself.[23] If you've had scans and other investigations and they've come back showing no significant damage yet you still feel considerable pain, this may be for you. I have had clients with chronic back pain observe significant benefits from this technique within several weeks of practice.

Regain Your Sex Life
Despite Pain

You may not find it surprising to learn that research proves people who have suffered from a painful problem for over 12 weeks are more likely to report a lack of sexual desire and satisfaction.[24] Being in pain is clearly not a turn-on for the sufferer. However, upon my search through the literature, I was surprised to learn that sex (more specifically, the chemicals released into our bloodstreams during intercourse) can have a significantly positive effect on pain.[25]

The mechanism for how this works is interesting. The endorphins (feel-good chemicals) released during sex interact with the opiate receptors in our brains in a similar way to drugs such as codeine or morphine. So, it appears there is a more enjoyable way to get similar positive pain-relieving benefits of these painkillers without suffering any of the nasty side effects.

There doesn't appear to be any research on a minimum frequency required to experience the positive effects of sex on pain, but as the painkilling effects seem to be transient, I would suggest that more is better!

In terms of practicality, however, when you're struggling with easily irritated pain, sex can be a logistical challenge. That's why I've done the research (just reading, I promise) to find out which positions might be the most comfortable, depending on what aggravates or eases your pain.

I have chosen to focus on the two problems that have the most negative impact on the sex lives of the clients I treat: hip pain and back pain. The following is based on literature published by Dr Stuart McGill, a leading back-pain researcher from Canada.

For Women with Back Pain

If your pain gets worse when you bend forward, you might want to try a variation of the "cowgirl" position—where you sit astride your partner, knees supported on the bed.

Instead of sitting upright in this position, you'll want to lean back and support your body weight by placing your hands on your partner's shins.

This position was shown to be one of the most comfortable for women who don't like to bend forward by researchers in the *European Spine Journal* in 2015.[26]

Alternatively, if you're fine bending forward but standing, walking and leaning back triggers your back pain, you might want to try a variation of the traditional "missionary" position, say the same researchers.

You can either go for the classic missionary position (lying on your back with knees bent, man on top), or a raunchier progression (your legs up, knees against his chest, man on top).

For Men with Back Pain

Gents, if your pain is worse when you bend forward, you will find most ease in a modified "cowgirl" position. This will involve your partner going on top, leaning forward, while you lie completely flat below her. This was the top recommended position for men who have difficulty flexing forward by Dr Stuart McGill, world-renowned back-pain researcher.[27]

If you are fine bending forward but have difficulty walking, standing, or leaning back because of back pain, you may have most luck lying on your side.

For this position, your partner should lie on her side, facing away from you, with her knees and hips bent up slightly. You will lie on your side pressed up against her back, with a similar body shape to her. This position will limit any "extension" movement from the lower back and should feel the most comfortable.

For Women with Hip Pain

With hip pain caused by arthritis or other aging changes, the hips lose significant mobility. This can make abduction (opening the legs) and rotation movements at the hip impossible. For this reason, we need to use a position that avoids these commonly restricted hip movements.

The main three limited movements tend to be:

- Internal rotation (turning the top of your thigh inward to "face" the other thigh)

- Abduction (spreading your legs apart)

- Flexion (bringing your knee up to your chest)

If we think technically about the sex positions that involve these movements, quite a few of the traditional positions might be ruled out.

Missionary position involves the woman abducting her legs. Cowgirl (woman on top) involves internal rotation to allow the legs to straddle either side of her partner.

There is, however, an effective position that limits all three of these actions while remaining comfortable for both parties. It is a type of modified all-fours position and this was reported to be most comfortable for the people with hip pain that I anonymously surveyed during my research for this book.

It involves the woman lying face down, her upper half supported by the bed, with her knees supported on the floor. If she shuffles her body forward, she can increase the angle between her thigh and her body to ease away from hip flexion, if this is an uncomfortable action. The man is then able to enter from behind, without the need for her to spread her legs into abduction.

For Men with Hip Pain

In traditional missionary, it is the thrusting of the man that provides the motion during sex. With hip pain, this thrusting action can be real agony for the man and lead to a poor experience all round, with considerable pain afterward.

If you are a male with hip pain and limited range of motion, the woman may have to start taking the lead in "female-dominant" positions. The cowgirl and reverse cowgirl (woman facing away) are great options in this case, as described above.

Journaling to Track Progress

If you want to make significant, positive changes in your life—whether that be to your health, your wellbeing or your relationships—there is one simple technique that can help you do so: tracking your progress. The premise behind this tip lies in the fact that if you can measure it, you can change it. As business management author Peter Drucker famously said, "What gets measured, gets managed."

Journaling has the potential to help us improve across many aspects of our lives. It can help us measure the results of our business ventures, track our health and fitness, hit goals more efficiently and organize our thoughts from an illogical mess into intelligible harmony.

I would recommend taking five minutes at the end of each day to track the following:

- The time you woke up.

- How you slept and how you felt when you woke up (on a 1 to 10 scale if this makes it easier).

- Brief description of the foods you ate for each meal (if you are making an effort to improve your health).

- What exercise you did that day.

- Some positive things that happened.

- Some negative things that you would like to improve.

Through the simple act of recording these things, you can actually improve them without even making a conscious effort.

This is because of something called the "Hawthorne effect": we are more likely to make better decisions when we know we are being observed, or when we are accountable, even if it is just writing it down at the end of the day.[28]

I've found that when I am tracking what I eat, for example, I make better choices. Why? It's not because I would rather eat healthy meals that day—it's because I know I have to write down whatever I put in my mouth (and the embarrassment of writing down "12 Maryland cookies" that evening is not something I wish to experience more than once).

This method is especially good for anyone who is a little overweight and struggles to shift the pounds. The sheer act of writing down what we eat each day helps to influence our choices and allows us to see where we might be going wrong.

Journaling is also great for anyone with chronic pain who really struggles to find positive moments in each day. Simply jotting down anything that made the day more bearable—visiting a friend, the touch of a loved one, a hot bath—will help you seek out these things in the future when you're suffering.

Play the "So What?" Game

It's incredible how our inner narrative can exacerbate even the most minor of inconveniences into something catastrophic.

Traffic notice goes up on the highway? Great, this will probably make me late. Everyone is going to think I can't manage my time effectively.

A missed call from work on my day off? It's probably bad news—what have I done wrong this time?

Incoming email marked URGENT from the bank? Maybe someone has cloned my card and emptied my account?

Can you relate?

Needless to say, on most of these occasions, the outcome is almost never as bad as we feared. All we have done with our worrying is dump cortisol into our systems, with no need for it to be there. As Mark Twain once said, "I've had a lot of worries in my life, most of which never happened."

By now we know that stress—especially low-level, persistent stress—can impact the body in a negative way, even amplifying painful experiences. So, what are we going to do about these harmful thinking patterns that serve no purpose but to make us worry needlessly?

If you've tried to "just stop thinking like that," then you'll know the harder you try, the worse it gets. But there is another way. I have been experimenting with a new method to control my own thought patterns and I have found that this really works to help me dissolve these unnecessary thoughts and avoid anxiety as a result. This method is based on a hybrid of two different philosophies that I have found personally useful.

The first is stoicism, a philosophy that began over 2,000 years ago in ancient Greece. It is designed to help us use the rational side of our brains to face adversity. Its most well-known practitioners include the Roman emperor Marcus Aurelius and Seneca the Younger.

The second philosophy is based on author Tim Ferriss's exercise called "Fear Setting." This is a tool that encourages us to face the worst things that could possibly happen to us head on—safely in our imagination. Ferriss asserts that much of the anxiety we face in our lives is due to our fear around what might go wrong in the future.[29] However, we are likely to be far less concerned about what might go wrong if we take the time to think about the consequences in advance and even put in mitigating steps to prevent them from impacting us so severely.

My iteration of these philosophies is called the "So What?" game and it's very simple. Every time you find a completely unfounded, disproportionate assumption about the future sneaking up on you like the ones in the example above, put your most rational hat on and ask yourself one question: "So what?"

So what if I AM three hours late?

In truth, it would be a minor inconvenience for the people I work with. The boss would probably understand—I'm never usually late so it's not like it's becoming a problem. Would it even be remembered tomorrow? Probably not.

So what if I HAVE made a serious error at work?

I know I am conscientious so I will deal with it with integrity and honesty. There might even be an opportunity here to learn something that will positively impact me in the future.

So what if someone HAS emptied my account?

In worries like this one, the consequences are obviously greater. However, the game still works. The way you go about remedying this is by detailing in your head the exact step-by-step plan you'd put in place if encountering this awful situation.

You'd probably first call the bank and let them know. You might have to survive for a few days without any bank cards while the fraud is investigated—but most of us would have someone willing to lend us a small amount of cash for a week until it's sorted, so that should be OK. Besides, bank fraud teams are so effective nowadays there would likely be ways to prove you've been the victim of theft.

Even if you don't get your money back—are you going to die? Probably not. You'll find someone to go and live with for a while until you're back on your feet. Sell the house, get a smaller place and start fresh. You could sell your car and other belongings if you needed to. Not ideal . . . but *you'd survive*—and proving this to yourself is the antidote to the very crux that anxiety stems from: worrying about preservation of your life. With this tool, it turns out there is a way that you can somewhat talk yourself out of this type of self-inflicted anxiety.

This technique can be a good tool to have in the toolbox for anyone struggling with low-level, day-to-day anxious thoughts. In the present day, that seems to be many of us, admittedly. I've found this tip very useful for when my thoughts start to run away with me; for the times when I feel overwhelmed by the possibility of terrible situations playing out in my head on repeat like a broken record.

I am not the first to employ this technique, as it would happen. In the ancient translated personal notes of Marcus Aurelius (Roman Emperor in 161 to 180 c.e.) in the book *Meditations*, arguably the most powerful man in the world makes notes to remind himself how he must truly examine his anxieties to get to the bottom of what they really are. Once you can imagine the ultimate outcome that you fear, and you are able to say "that really wouldn't be so bad," anxieties tend to abate.

Give it a try next time you feel helpless or despairing. What have you got to lose in those moments?

How to Keep the Mind Young

It is a fact that the human brain changes as we age.[30] It would be possible to see physical changes in the brain of a senior when compared to the brain of someone thirty years younger. This matches up to most people's lived experience, too. Many people report feeling a little less "sharp" in their more senior years. However, while many of these changes are unavoidable to some extent, a decline in cognition may not necessarily be inevitable.

Two of the most common mental health problems in the later stages of life are dementia and depression. The World Health Organization estimates that 5 percent of people over sixty suffer from dementia, while 7 percent suffer from depression; although these problems may be vastly under-reported.[31] Dementia is a syndrome that primarily affects the older adult but it is not a natural part of aging. Contrary to popular belief, getting names wrong from time to time and occasionally losing the keys are not early signs of dementia. However, significant confusion and persistent forgetfulness can be.

Depression can affect anyone of any age, but the rate at which it affects the senior population is alarming. There are many factors that contribute to why this might be the case. One factor is loneliness.[32] Being lonely is a leading factor in depression. Loss of mobility and pain can also be a contributing cause, as well as loss of loved ones (which is, again, more likely with age).

Thankfully, even though we cannot always prevent these conditions, both crippling problems can be staved off to a degree by our behavior. You may have read in the media how it's possible to slow down the mental aging process by keeping the mind active and nimble. There's a lot of truth in this claim and experts believe we should exercise the brain, just as we exercise the body. So, mental exercise is important—but how do we effectively exercise the mind to stave off the effects of aging as much as possible?

Here are a few ways to keep your mind young, ward off depression and minimize your chances of dementia in your advancing years:

Mental Gymnastics

Contrary to popular belief, the act of solving puzzles—such as the popular numbers game Sudoku—has never actually been shown to prevent dementia or cognitive decline. While the puzzles may improve overall cognition, they probably won't prevent dementia, a study carried out at the University of Aberdeen suggests.[33] Instead, the researchers recommend three different forms of brain exercise that may have more potential for staving off dementia: reading, playing board games and playing a musical instrument. These enjoyable yet mentally challenging tasks are hypothesized to slow down the rate of "brain atrophy" that occurs with age and help to keep the mind young. How does playing a board game differ to solving a puzzle, you might ask? It could be in the fact that another person is involved in the task. Being sociable has been shown to have a hugely positive impact on brain function in older adults.[34]

Treat the Body, Treat the Mind

There is a wealth of evidence to suggest that exercise can act as a protective factor for both dementia and depression in advancing years.[35] People who exercise are generally happier and have better quality of life.[36] A healthy body really does stimulate a healthy mind through a combination of physical and psychological factors. On the physical side, blood pressure, lipid profiles and blood sugar levels are all improved in people who take daily exercise.[37] Having these three markers running amok would certainly increase one's risk of suffering dementia, as well as significant health events like a stroke. The fallout of an incident like a heart attack or a stroke is often long-term disability, which may lead to depression in many cases. Keep your heart healthy, your lungs in good shape and your muscles strong, and you'll be giving not just your body but your mind as well the best possible chance.

Stick the Kettle on

While the neuro-protective qualities of tea are still up for debate, there's one thing that has been shown to have a significant effect on mental health in later life—and that is your social circle. Maintaining good links between friends and family, with regular and enjoyable contact, has been proven to stimulate the mind and reduce the risks of dementia and depression alike.[38] Simply having a catch-up with a friend is enough to get your daily quota of human contact—but there are bonus points up for grabs if you engage in a fun activity with that friend, too. Playing board games, taking a long walk, or going to a museum are all preferable to simply sitting at home, as you'll get the mental stimulation and exercise associated with these activities at the same time as the social benefits.

Avoid the Deadly Sins

Smoking has been shown to be associated with an increased risk of dementia later in life, as well as a multitude of other unwanted health problems.[39] Do your mind and body a favor and quit, or at least cut down, if you're a smoker. As for drinking, pay some attention to the government guidelines that set a clear limit for our weekly alcohol intake and see how you measure up. If you regularly exceed this limit, it's probably a good idea to cut back.

Spend Some Time with Mother Nature

There is a growing body of research, relevant to people of all ages and for a variety of health conditions, that shows just how beneficial it is to spend time in the great outdoors. There's evidence to show that work productivity goes up just by putting plants in offices.[40] We can significantly reduce the risk of depression just by taking long walks in the woods or on the beach.[41] Taking time to appreciate the beauty of the outdoors is a wonderful way to stay healthy in both body and mind. Be sure to schedule some time for yourself to spend in nature in the next few days and take note of how you feel after—you may find it so valuable that it becomes a non-negotiable!

Create a Healthy Habit

How do some people seemingly find it so easy to eat well, go to the gym day after day and stay in amazing shape all year round?

Are they lucky? Do they simply have good genes? Is it because they spend more money on their health than others?

I would argue that, in most cases, it's none of these things. The people who are successful with their health have simply developed healthy habits. And habits are the key to long-term success.

There is research to suggest that we have a limited amount of willpower to use in any given day.[42] Willpower is finite; by resisting temptation over and over again, we run the risk of "willpower fatigue." When we reach this point of fatigue, just like having a weakened immune system, we are much more likely to make bad decisions that lead to poor health.

Every time you open the fridge and have to make a choice about what to eat, you're depleting your willpower reserves. Every time you visit the supermarket and walk past the ice cream section, you're using up willpower. Every time you put on your sneakers, even though it's raining, you're burning through even more of your precious willpower.

My theory is that if we have to make a decision—"shall I, shan't I?"—in each of these situations, we've *already* lost. There's only a certain number of times we can overcome our desire to do the easy thing before we succumb to the instantly gratifying choice of staying on the sofa, ordering a takeaway, or picking up that ice cream.

So, if the act of making these decisions makes it harder for us to stay healthy, what are we supposed to do? The answer is simple: *we avoid making these decisions altogether.*

At first glance, that recommendation sounds ridiculous—but if you think a little more about it, it makes perfect sense. The people who are successful with making healthy decisions, day after day, do so not because they have superior willpower but because they put themselves into a position where they *automatically* make the right choice, without having to consider it.

How do you make the right choice become the automatic option? You simply have to make it far easier TO make the right choice than NOT to make it!

Let me give you some examples: if you're determined to go for a walk tomorrow morning, even when it's cold, dark and wet, make it as easy as possible for your future self by preparing the night before. Start by laying out all your walking clothes on the end of your bed, including an extra layer in case it's even colder than expected. Hide away all your shoes, except your walking boots. Now, before you go to bed, set your alarm out of your reach when you're in bed. Tomorrow, when your alarm goes off, it'll be far easier to get up and put on your walking clothes than it will be to put them all away again and find something different to wear.

Another example I can give you represents a brilliant way to cut junk food out of your life. As it turns out, you can make healthy choices the easiest thing in the world. As humans, we have a tendency to make lifestyle choices based on convenience. This is one of the reasons why gaining weight is so easy in the first place: fattening, sugary foods are also the ones that are cheapest and easiest to get your hands on. But what would happen if you made those foods the most difficult to acquire, and healthier foods the most convenient option? Do you think you'd make better choices?

One way to do this is to be sure to eat a satiating meal before you go for your weekly shop (we make worse food purchasing decisions when hungry), so you find it much easier to buy only healthy foods and leave your usual temptations on the shelf. Even better, write a strict list before you go, leaving out any junk food. When you get home, discard or ask a friend to remove the sugary, fattening foods that currently live in your kitchen and pantry so you're left with nothing in the house except healthy food. The third part of this process is to ensure you make a small amount extra of any healthy meal and store it in the fridge, so you have instantly accessible (yet healthy) snacks should you get hungry between meals.

When the cravings arise—and they will—you'll have a choice: eat the pre-prepared healthy food . . . or get your wallet, get in your car, drive all the way to the shop and buy a sugary snack. Eight or nine times out of ten, you'll be likely to opt for the healthier choice out of sheer convenience. In this way, you don't even need to think of this process as "being on a diet." You're still allowed the naughty food, after all; you just have to work a little harder for it!

By making the right choice the *default* choice, you make it much easier for your brain to shortcut the decision-making process. These little choices all add up, and it gets easier as time goes on. After you make the right choice hundreds of times in a row, a habit is formed. And when a habit is formed, it becomes more of an effort to go against your healthy habit than it does to follow it from here on.

Conclusion

The human body is a complex and wonderful creation. The astonishing scale of the tiny but significant chemical reactions that occur within our bodies every day to keep us alive is enough to spend a lifetime wondering over. Within this plethora of reactions is the human ability to feel pain. While it may not feel like a blessing at times, pain is as valuable and important a sensation as touch, smell or taste.

The Power of Pain

Pain guides us every single day of our lives.

Pain is the reason you instinctively react to pull your hand away from a knife blade. Pain is the driving force behind the muscles in your ankle contracting to prevent an ankle sprain, before your consciousness can even begin to process that action.

And, on another level, emotional pain moves us to take action. It motivates us to make changes. If we didn't get uncomfortable sometimes, we wouldn't have the drive to accomplish anything significant.

Without certain types of pain, we would not survive for long. There are people who are born without the same ability to process pain as the rest of us, with a condition called congenital insensitivity to pain. They have turned out not to be very successful in terms of survival; without the feedback mechanisms that pain provides, many of them die in their twenties by taking ridiculously dangerous risks, unrestrained by the threat of severe pain.[43]

However, pain isn't always necessary. In this book, I've tried to provide you with some solutions to solve the nagging, painful problems that get in the way of living your life to its fullest. Hopefully, you've learned something along the way that you can now apply to your own life.

If you aren't suffering from a painful problem, I hope you've still found great value in the recommendations I've presented to you about how we should be living to prolong life as best we can. We only get one chance at this game of life, and turning small daily actions into healthy habits is the way to ensure your health for the years ahead of you.

Not Just the Physical

Of course, as we've discussed in this book, it isn't just your physical body that you must pay attention to. The mind is as important, and strategies that improve your mental health and wellbeing are as valuable as physical exercise when it comes to staying fit and able in your advancing years.

My challenge to you upon completion of this book is to simply remain aware of the areas of your body and mind that might need a little work to remain healthy as you grow older. Did you struggle to complete the Nine at Ninety? Do you have aches or pains that haven't resolved over the last few months? Are you feeling lonely or in need of some mental stimulation? If you answered "yes" to any of these questions, you know exactly where you need to start in order to get, and stay, physically and mentally healthy.

An important thing to remember as you spend more time working on your health is that you're not alone in this. There are people who have dedicated their careers to helping others achieve these (often overwhelming) goals of becoming or staying healthy despite their years working against them. I am one such individual. So, if you're in Surrey and would like a helping hand, you'd be more than welcome to stop by for a chat and a coffee where my friendly team can show you exactly what you need to do to get you fit, healthy and mobile again.

Simply head to our website (you can find the address in the Resources section) if you'd like to learn more about how you can get some help to achieve your goals.

If you're not in my area, but would still like some help, you can find our popular YouTube channel by searching "HT Physio" on YouTube. There are hundreds of videos on my channel—completely free—which will show you exercises, tips and strategies for solving painful problems and improving your health. You can find links to my YouTube channel in the Resources section.

If you want something more in-depth than our YouTube videos, we have a special program for those who are serious about improving their strength, mobility and independence. Lifelong Mobility is my online program where I walk you through my best exercise routines for improving every aspect of your physical health. Learn more about the Lifelong Mobility™ program in the Resources section.

Biggest Take-Home Message

If I had to distill the take-home message from this book down to one sentence, it would be this: Don't feel as though you have to accept aches, pains, poor mobility, "slowing down," becoming lonely and missing out on the things you love as just a part of getting older!

There is no need for it to be that way for most people reading this, and there are usually things that can be done to improve your situation, even if you've initially been told you just need to "accept it" as a fact of life. I am an advocate for second opinions; it's something we try to do for people every day in my clinic. So, if nothing else, please take the hope that I'm trying to pass on to you from these pages—that growing older doesn't have to represent a slow decline in health and mobility. People regularly come into my clinic and say, "It's no fun getting old," but I like to encourage them to see the positives they can take from their advancing years. Experience, wisdom and patience are all virtues we gain with each passing year, and I'm sure you are no different.

One of the greatest gifts you can give to yourself in your fifties and beyond is the gift of physical activity. Staying active has been shown to protect your heart, muscles and even your brain. It's a common occurrence to hear a doctor remark that if there was a pill that could give us the benefits of exercise, people would be queuing round the corner to get a prescription. Luckily, we don't need to wait until a wonder drug is invented when there are so many different forms of exercise and activity readily available to us; just pick one that works for you. Summoning the willpower to get started is genuinely the biggest hurdle, but the more you flex that hypothetical muscle, the stronger it gets. Keep making the right choices for your body, day after day, and the little decisions all add up.

As for following diets and nutrition plans, don't overcomplicate it. Try to make better choices, one by one, and take advantage of our tendency to take the most convenient option available to us (*see also pages 394–396*). If you're looking to shed a few pounds, this may involve putting obstacles between you and junk food.

Armed with the information and guidance in this book, you should have a better chance of remaining healthy and injury-free, which will directly improve your quality of life and the lives of your family. One thing that my clients report worrying about perhaps more than anything else is that their family may have to suffer in order to take care of them as they become sick or less mobile. By staying fit, well and injury-free, you'll not only be giving yourself an incredible gift, but you'll also be doing the same for your family. Imagine having a few extra years to play with the grandchildren that you otherwise wouldn't have had: can you put a price on that?

References

Part One: Cracking the Fundamentals

1 Matthews, C.E., et al. (2019). "Amount and intensity of leisure–time physical activity and lower cancer risk." *J. Clin Oncol.* [ePub ahead of print.]

2 Wange, R. and Holsinger, R.M.D. (2018). "Exercise-induced brain-derived neurotrophic factor expression: therapeutic implications for Alzheimer's dementia." *Ageing Research Review.* 48: 109–21.

Part Two: Head, Neck and Shoulders

1 Rasmussen, B.K., et al. (1991). "Epidemiology of headache in a general population—a prevalence study." *J Clin Epidemiol.* https://pubmed.ncbi.nlm.nih.gov/1941010/ [Accessed 14 June 2024]

2 Shaik, M.M. and Gan, S.H. (2015). "Vitamin supplementation as possible prophylactic treatment against migraine with aura and menstrual migraine." *Biomed Res Int.* https://pubmed.ncbi.nlm.nih.gov/25815319/ [Accessed 7 June 2024]

3 Määttä J, et al. (2022). "Lower thoracic spine extension mobility is associated with higher intensity of thoracic spine pain." *J. Man. Manip. Ther.* 30(5): 300–8.

4 Wang, K., et al. (2013). "Risk factors in idiopathic adhesive capsulitis: a case control study." *J. Shoulder Elbow Surg.* 22(7): e24–e29.

5 Malavolta, E.A., et al. (2018). "Asian ethnicity: a risk factor for adhesive capsulitis?" *Rev. Bras Ortop.* 53(5): 602–6.

6 Franz, A., et al. (2019). "Conservative treatment of frozen shoulder." *Unfallchirurg.* 122(12): 934–40.

7 Pieters, L., et al. (2019). "An update of systematic reviews examining the effectiveness of conservative physiotherapy interventions for subacromial shoulder pain." *JOSPT.* 1–33.

8 Lawrence, R.L., et al. (2019). "Asymptomatic rotator cuff tears." *JBJS Rev.* 7(6): 9.

9 Horsley, I., et al. (2016). "Do changes in hand grip strength correlate with shoulder rotator cuff function?" *Shoulder Elbow.* 8(2): 124–9.

10 Carroll, L.J., et al. (2008). "Course and prognostic factors for neck pain in whiplash-associated disorders (WAD): results of the Bone and Joint Decade 2000–2010 Task Force on Neck Pain and Its Associated Disorders." *Spine.* 33(4): 83–92.

Part Three: Wrists, Elbows and Hands

1 van den Heuvel, S.G., et al. (2003). "Effects of software programs stimulating regular breaks and exercises on work-related neck and upper-limb disorders." *Scand. J. Work Environ. Health.* 29(2): 106–16.

2 Kim, T.N. and Choi, K.M. (2013). "Sarcopenia: definition, epidemiology, and pathophysiology." *J. Bone Metab.* 20(1): 1–10.

3 Moore, D.R. (2014). "Keeping older muscle 'young' through dietary protein and physical activity." *Adv. Nutr.* 5(5): 599–607.

4 Bohannon, R.W. (2019). "Grip Strength: An Indispensable Biomarker For Older Adults." *Clin. Interv. Aging.* 1(14): 1681–91.

Part Four: Back Pain and Sciatica

1 National Institute of Neurological Disorders and Stroke (2020). https://www.ninds.nih.gov/sites/default/files/migrate-documents/low_back_pain_20-ns-5161_march_2020_508c.pdf [Accessed 7 June 2024]

2 Eshed, I., Lidar, M. (2017). "MRI findings of the sacroiliac joints in patients with low back pain: Alternative diagnosis to inflammatory sacroiliitis." *Isr. Med. Assoc. J.* 19(11): 666–9.

3 Assaker, R. and Zairi, F. (2015). "Failed back surgery syndrome: to re-operate or not to re-operate? A retrospective review of patient selection and failures." *Neurochirurgie.* 61: 77–82.

4 Brinjikji, W., et al. (2015). "Systematic literature review of imaging features of spinal degeneration in asymptomatic populations." *AJNR Am. J. Neuroradiol.* 36(4): 811–16.

5 Bernstein, I.A., et al. (2021). "Low back pain and sciatica: summary of NICE guidance." *BMJ.* 2017 Jan 6; 356: i6748.

6 Barbosa, A.B.M., et al. (2019). "Sciatic nerve and its variations: is it possible to associate them with piriformis syndrome?" *Arq. Neuropsiquiatr.* 77(9): 646–53.

7 Berthelot, J.M., et al. (2018). "Stretching of roots contributes to the pathophysiology of radiculopathies." *Joint Bone Spine.* 85(1): 41–5.

8 Strauss, A.T., et al. (2019). "The effect of total motion release on functional movement screen composite scores: A randomised controlled trial." *J. Sport Rehabil.* Dec: 1–9.

9 Sheahan, P.J., et al. (2016). "The effect of rest break schedule on acute low back pain development in pain and non-pain developers during seated work." *Appl. Ergon.* 53: 64–70.

10 Daneshmandi H., et al. (2017). "Adverse effects of prolonged sitting behavior on the general health of office workers." *J. Lifestyle Med.* 7(2): 69–75.

11 Szczygiel, E., et al. (2017). "Musculo-skeletal and pulmonary effects of sitting position—a systematic review." *Ann. Agric. Environ. Med.* 24(1): 8–12.

12 De Blaiser, C., et al. (2018). "Is core stability a risk factor for lower extremity injuries in an athletic population? A systematic review." *Phys. Ther. Sport.* 30: 48–56.

13 Kendall, J.C., et al. (2014). "Foot posture, leg length discrepancy and low back pain—their relationship and clinical management using foot orthoses—an overview." *Foot (Edinburgh).* 24(2): 75–80.

14 Resende, R.A., et al. (2019). "Effects of foot pronation on the lower limb sagittal plane biomechanics during gait." *Gait Posture.* 68: 130–35.

15 Unver, B., et al. (2019). "Effects of short-foot exercises on foot posture, pain, disability, and plantar pressure in pen planus." *J. Sport Rehabil.* 16: 1–5.

16 Shi J., et al. (2023). "Effects of breathing exercises on low back pain in clinical: A systematic review and meta-analysis." *Complement. Ther. Med.* 79: 102993

17 Urfy M.Z. and Suarez, J.I. (2014). "Breathing and the nervous system." *Handb. Clin. Neurol.* 119: 241–50.

Part Five: Hips and Knees

1 Ebert J.R., et al. (2017). "A systematic review of rehabilitation exercises to progressively load the gluteus medius." *J. Sport Rehabil.* 26(5): 418–36.

2 Alaia, M.J., et al. (2015). "The utility of plan radiographs in the initial evaluation of knee pain amongst sports medicine patients." *Knee Surg. Sports Traumatol. Arthrosc.* 23(8): 2213–17.

3 de Oliveira Silva, D., et al. (2018). "Implications of knee crepitus to the overall clinical presentation of women with and without patellofemoral pain." *Physical Therapy in Sport.* 33: 89–95.

4   Glaviano, N.R. and Saliba, S. (2019). "Differences in gluteal and quadriceps muscle activation during weight-bearing exercises between female subjects with and without patellofemoral pain." *J. Strength Cond Res.* [epub ahead of print].

5   Schiphof, D., et al. (2014). "Crepitus is a first indication of patellofemoral osteoarthritis (and not of tibiofemoral arthritis)." *Osteoarthritis Cartilage.* 22(5): 631–8.

6   Jibri, Z., et al. (2019). "Patellar maltracking: an update on the diagnosis and treatment strategies." *Insights Imaging.* 10(1): 65.

7   Li, J.S., et al. (2019). "Weight loss changed gait kinematics in individuals with obesity and knee pain." *Gait Posture.* 68: 461–5.

8   Mun, F., et al. (2015). "Kinematic relationship between rotation of lumbar spine and hip joints during golf swing in professional golfers." https://pubmed.ncbi.nlm.nih.gov/25971396/ [Accessed 7 June 2024]

9   MacDonald, K.V., et al. (2014). "Symptom onset, diagnosis and management of osteoarthritis." *Health Rep.* 25(9): 10–17.

10 Klassbo, M., et al. (2003). "Examination of passive ROM and capsular patterns in the hip." *Physiother. Res. Int.* 8(1): 1–12.

11 Park, K.N., et al. (2016). "Effects of motor control exercise vs muscle stretching exercise on reducing compensatory lumbopelvic motions and low back pain: a randomised trial." *J. Manipulative Physiol. Ther.* 39(8): 576–85.

12 Gov.uk (2022). "Falls: applying all our health." https://www.gov.uk/government/publications/ falls-applying-all-our-health/falls-applying-all-our-health#:~:text=unaddressed%20fall%20 hazards%20in%20the,2%20billion%20of%20 this%20sum [Accessed 7 June 2024]

13 Sherrington, C. and Tiedemann, A. (2015). "Physiotherapy in the prevention of falls in older people." *J. Physiother.* 61: 54–60.

14 Negendank, W.G., et al. (1990). "Magnetic resonance imaging of meniscal degeneration in asymptomatic knees." *J. Orthop. Res.* 8(3): 311–20.

15 Jin, X., et al. (2016). "Longitudinal associations between adiposity and change in knee pain: Tasmanian older adult cohort study." *Semin. Arthritis Rheum.* 45(5): 564–9.

16 Hicks-Little, C.A., et al. (2016). "The relationship between early-stage knee osteoarthritis and lower-extremity alignment, joint laxity, and subjective scores of pain, stiffness and function." *J. Sport Rehabil.* 25(3): 213–18.

17 Lee, J.Y., et al. (2018). "Lower leg muscle mass relates to knee pain in patients with knee osteoarthritis." *Int. J. Rheum. Dis.* 21(1): 126–33.

18 Guedes, V., Castro, J.P., Brito, I. (2018). "Topical capsaicin for pain in osteoarthritis: A literature review." *Rheumatol. Clin.* 14(1): 40–5.

19 Hurley M., Dickson K., Hallett R., et al. (2018). "Exercise interventions and patient beliefs for people with hip, knee or hip and knee osteoarthritis: a mixed methods review." *Cochrane Database Syst. Rev.* 4(4): CD010842.

20 Torres, A., et al. (2018). "Greater trochanteric pain syndrome and gluteus medius and minimus tendinosis: nonsurgical treatment." *Pain Management.* 8(1): 45–55.

21 Ganderton, C., et al. (2017). "A comparison of gluteus medius, gluteus minimus and tensor fascia latae muscle activation during gait in post-menopausal women with and without greater trochanteric pain syndrome." *J. Electromyogr. Kinesiol.* 33: 39–47.

22 Paluska, S.A. and McKeag, D.B. (2000). "Knee braces: current evidence and clinical recommendations for their use." *American Family Physician.* 61(2): 411–18.

23 Jensen, S.B., et al. (2010). "Is it possible to reduce the knee joint compression force during level walking with hiking poles?" *Scandinavian Journal of Medicine & Science in Sports.* 21(6): 195–200.

24 Muché J.A. (2003). "Efficacy of therapeutic ultrasound treatment of a meniscus tear in a severely disabled patient: a case report." *Arch. Phys. Med. Rehabil.* 84(10): 1558–9.

Part Six: Feet and Ankles

1   de Jonge, S., van den Berg, C., de Vos, R.J., et al. (2011). "Incidence of midportion Achilles tendinopathy in the general population." *Br. J. Sports Med.* 45: 1026–8.

2   Chang, H.J., et al. (2010). "Achilles Tendinopathy." *JAMA.* 303(2): 188.

3   Roche, A.J. and Calder, J.D.F. (2013). "Achilles tendinopathy: A review of the current concepts of treatment." *Bone Joint Journal.* 95: 1299–307.

4   Redmond, A.C., et al. (2008). "Normative values for the Foot Posture Index." *J. Foot Ankle Res.* 1, 6.

5   Gross, K.D., et al. (2011). "Association of flat feet with knee pain and cartilage damage in older adults." *Arthritis Care Res.* 63: 937–44.

6   Sachithanandam, V. and Joseph, B. (1995). "The influence of footwear on the prevalence of flat foot. A survey of 1846 skeletally mature persons." *J. Bone Joint Surg. Br. Mar*; 77(2): 254–7. PMID: 7706341.

7   Latey, P.J., et al. (2014). "Relationship between intrinsic foot muscle weakness and pain: a systematic review." *J. Foot Ankle Res.* 7: 51.

8   Hertel, J. (2000). "Functional instability following lateral ankle sprain." *Sports Med.* 29: 361.

9   Kibler, W. B., et al. (1991). "Functional biomechanical deficits in running athletes with plantar fasciitis." *AJSM.* 19(1): 66–71.

10 Torg, J.S., et al. (1987). "Overuse injuries in sport: the foot." *Clinics in Sports Medicine.* 6(2): 291–320.

11 McClinton, S., et al. (2016). "Impaired foot plantar flexor muscle performance in individuals with plantar heel pain and association with foot orthosis use." *JOSPT.* 46(8): 681–8.

12 Cychosz, C.C., et al. (2015). "Gastrocnemius recession for foot and ankle conditions in adults: Evidence-based recommendations." *Foot Ankle Surg.* Jun; 21(2): 77–85.

13 Bolívar, Y.A, et al. (2013). "Relationship between tightness of the posterior muscles of the lower limb and plantar fasciitis." *Foot Ankle Int.* Jan; 34(1): 42–8.

14 Clinghan, R., et al. (2008). "Do you get value for money when you buy an expensive pair of running shoes?" *Br. J. Sports Med.* Mar; 42(3): 189–93.

Part Seven: Whole-Body Health

1   Marsolais, D. and Frenette, J. (2005). "Inflammation and tendon healing." *Medicine Sciences*: M/S. Feb; 21(2): 181–6.

2   Izaola, O., et al. (2015). "Inflammation and obesity (lipoinflammation)." *Nutr. Hosp.* Jun 1; 31(6): 2352–8.

3   Butkowski, E.G. and Jelinek, H.F. (2017). "Hyperglycaemia, oxidative stress and inflammatory markers." *Redox. Rep. Nov*; 22(6): 257–64.

4   Li, M., et al. (2018). "Pro- and anti-inflammatory effects of short chain fatty acids on immune and endothelial cells." *Eur. J. Pharmacol.* Jul 15; 831: 52–9.

5   Tibuakuu, M., et al. (2017). "The association between cigarette smoking and inflammation: The Genetic Epidemiology Network of Arteriopathy (GENOA) study." *PLoS One.* 12(9).

6   Lancaster T. and Stead, L.F. (2017). "Individual behavioural counselling for smoking cessation." *Cochrane Database of Systematic Reviews*, Issue 3. Art. No.: CD001292.

7   Imhof, A., et al. (2001). "Effect of alcohol consumption on systemic markers of inflammation." *Lancet* 357 (9258), 763–7.

8   Elks, C.M. and Francis, J. (2010). "Central adiposity, systemic inflammation, and the metabolic syndrome." *J. Curr. Hypertens Rep.* 12: 99.

9   Aoki, K.C. and Mayrovitz, H.N. (2022). "Utility of a body shape index parameter in predicting cardiovascular disease risks." *Cureus*. Apr 6; 14(4): e23886.

10 Gunathilake, K.D.P.P., et al. (2018). "In vitro anti-inflammatory properties of selected green leafy vegetables." *Biomedicines*. Nov 19; 6(4). pii: E107.

11 Korrapati, D., et al. (2019). "Coconut oil consumption improves fat-free mass, plasma HDL-cholesterol and insulin sensitivity in healthy men with normal BMI compared to peanut oil." *Clin. Nutr. Dec*; 38(6): 2889–99.

12 Wongwarawipat, T., et al. (2018). "Olive oil-related anti-inflammatory effects on atherosclerosis: potential clinical implications." *Endocr. Metab. Immune Disord. Drug Targets*. 18(1): 51–62.

13 Artemis P. Simopoulos (2002). "Omega-3 fatty acids in inflammation and autoimmune diseases." *Journal of the American College of Nutrition*. 21(6): 495–505.

14 The Association of UK Dieticians (2021). "Where do Omega-3 fats come from?" https://www.bda.uk.com/resource/omega-3.html [Accessed 21 May 2024]

15 Lisa, S., et al. (2011). Effect of blueberry ingestion on natural killer cell counts, oxidative stress, and inflammation prior to and after 2.5 h of running." *Applied Physiology, Nutrition, and Metabolism*. 36: 976–84

16 Murphy, M.H., et al. (2002). "Accumulating brisk walking for fitness, cardiovascular risk, and psychological health." *Med Sci Sports Exerc*. 34(9): 1468–74.

17 De Luca, C. and Olefsky, J.M. (2007). "Inflammation and insulin resistance." *FEBS Lett*. Jan 9; 582(1): 97–105.

18 Charest, J. and Grandner, M.A. (2020). "Sleep and athletic performance: Impacts on physical performance, mental performance, injury risk and recovery, and mental health." *Sleep Med. Clin*. Mar; 15(1): 41–57.

19 St-Onge, M.P., et al. (2016). "Sleep duration and quality: Impact on lifestyle behaviors and cardiometabolic health: A scientific statement from the American Heart Association." *Circulation*. 134(18): e367–e386.

20 Åkerstedt, T., et al. (2021). "Sleep duration and mortality, influence of age, retirement, and occupational group." *J. Sleep Res*. 2022 Jun; 31(3): e13512.

21 Kocsis, M. (2023). "What is hormone imbalance?" https://balancemyhormones.co.uk/what-is-hormone-imbalance/ [Accessed 21 May 2024]

22 Guthrie, J.R., et al. (2003). "Central abdominal fat and endogenous hormones during the menopausal transition." *Fertility and Sterility*. 79(6): 1335–40.

23 Leproult, R. and Van Cauter, E. (2010). "Role of sleep and sleep loss in hormonal release and metabolism." *Endocr*. Dev. 17: 11–21.

24 Dumoulin, C., et al. (2014). "Pelvic floor muscle training versus no treatment, or inactive control treatments, for urinary incontinence in women." *Cochrane Database of Systematic Reviews*, Issue 5.

25 Morley, J.E., et al. (1997). "Longitudinal changes in testosterone, luteinizing hormone, and follicle-stimulating hormone in healthy older men." *Metabolism*. 46(4): 410–13.

26 Shores, M.M., et al. (2012). "Testosterone treatment and mortality in men with low testosterone levels." *J. Clin. Endocrinol Metab*. 97(6): 2050–2058.

27 Pilz, S., et al. (2011). "Effect of vitamin D supplementation on testosterone levels in men." *Horm. Metab. Res*. 43(3): 223–5.

28 MacLaughlin, J. and Holick, M.F. (1985). "Aging decreases the capacity of human skin to produce vitamin D3." *J. Clin. Invest*. 76(4): 1536–8.

29 Littlejohns, T.J., et al. (2014). "Vitamin D and the risk of dementia and Alzheimer's disease." *Neurology*. 83(10): 920–928.

30   Kraemer, W.J. et al. (1999). "Effects of heavy-resistance training on hormonal response patterns in younger vs. older men." *J. Appl Physiol.* 87(3): 982–92.

31   Hunter, G.R., et al. (2004). "Effects of resistance training on older adults." *Sports Med.* 34, 329–48.

32   Layne, J.E. and Nelson, M.E. (1999). "The effects of progressive resistance training on bone density: a review." *Medicine & Science in Sports & Exercise.* 31(1): 25–30.

33   Hudec, S. and Camacho, P. (2013). "Secondary causes of osteoporosis." *Endocrine Practice.* January, 19(1): 120–8.

34   Melton, L.J., III, Chrischilles, E.A., Cooper, C., Lane, A.W. and Riggs, B.L. (2005). "How many women have osteoporosis?" *J. Bone Miner. Res.* 20: 886–892.

35   Pacifici, R. (1996). "Estrogen, cytokines, and pathogenesis of postmenopausal osteoporosis." *J. Bone Miner. Res.* 11: 1043–51.

36   Holick, M.F. (2004). "Vitamin D: importance in the prevention of cancers, type 1 diabetes, heart disease, and osteoporosis." *AJCN.* 79(3): 362–71.

37   Chen, Z., et al. (2022). "Effects of zinc, magnesium, and iron ions on bone tissue engineering." *ACS Biomater. Sci. Eng.* Jun 13; 8(6): 2321–35.

38   Piuri, G., et al. (2021). "Magnesium in obesity, metabolic syndrome, and type 2 diabetes." *Nutrients.* 13(2): 320.

39   Palermo, A., et al. (2017). "Vitamin K and osteoporosis: Myth or reality?" *Metabolism.* 70: 57–71.

40   Newman, A.B., et al. (2006). "Strength, but not muscle mass, is associated with mortality in the health, aging and body composition study cohort." *J. Gerontol. Series A,* 61(1): 72–7.

41   Wickham, C., et al. (1989). "Muscle strength, activity, housing and the risk of falls in elderly people." *Age and Ageing.* 18(1): 47–51.

42   Schilke, J. M., et al. (1996). "Effects of muscle-strength training on the functional status of patients with osteoarthritis of the knee joint." *Nursing Research.* March–April, 45(2): 68–72.

43   Cunningham, J.J. (1982). "Body composition and resting metabolic rate: the myth of feminine metabolism." *AJCN.* 36(4): 721–6.

44   Lachman, M.E., et al. (2006). "The effects of strength training on memory in older adults." *JAPA.* 14(1): 59–73.

45   Hickson, R.C., et al. (1980). Strength training effects on aerobic power and short–term endurance. Medicine and Science in Sports and Exercise. 12(5): 336–9.

46   Rainville, J., et al. (2004). Exercise as a treatment for chronic low back pain. The Spine Journal. 4(1): 106–15.

47   O'Connor, P.J., et al. (2010). Mental health benefits of strength training in adults. American Journal of Lifestyle Medicine. 4(5): 377–96.

48   Mayer, F., et al. (2011). The intensity and effects of strength training in the elderly. Dtsch. Arztebl. Int. 108(21): 359–64.

49   Baum, J.I., et al. (2016). "Protein Consumption and the Elderley: What Is the Optimal Level of Intake?" https://www.ncbi.nlm.nih.gov/pmc/articles/PMC4924200/ [Accessed 8 June 2024]

50   Sawitzke, A.D., et al. (2010). "Clinical efficacy and safety of glucosamine, chondroitin sulphate, their combination, celecoxib or placebo taken to treat osteoarthritis of the knee: 2–year results from GAIT." *Ann. Rheum. Dis.* 69(8): 1459–64.

51   Henrotin, Y., et al. (2014). "What is the current status of chondroitin sulfate and glucosamine for the treatment of knee osteoarthritis?" *Maturitas.* 78(3): 184–7.

52   Cooke, R. (2017). "Sleep should be prescribed: what those late nights out could be costing you." https://www.theguardian.com/lifeandstyle/2017/sep/24/why-lack-of-sleep-health-worst-enemy-matthew-walker-why-we-sleep [Accessed 21 May 2024]

53 *The Jordan Harbinger Show*, podcast episode 126. "Matthew Walker, Unlocking the power of sleep and dreams." https://www.jordanharbinger.com/matthew-walker-unlocking-the-power-of-sleep-and-dreams/ [Accessed 21 May 2024]

54 Chellappa, S.L., et al. (2013). "Acute exposure to evening blue-enriched light impacts on human sleep." *J. Sleep Res.* 22: 573–80.

55 Murphy, P.J. and Campbell, S.S. (1997). "Night-time drop in body temperature: A physiological trigger for sleep onset." *Sleep.* 20(7): 505–11.

56 Baniassadi, A., et al. (2023). "Night-time ambient temperature and sleep in community-dwelling older adults." *Sci. Total Environ.* 899: 165623.

57 Sutanto, C.N. et al. (2022). "The impact of tryptophan supplementation on sleep quality: a systematic review, meta-analysis, and meta-regression." *Nutr. Rev.* 80(2): 306–16.

58 Minich, D.M., et al. (2022). "Is melatonin the 'Next Vitamin D'?: A review of emerging science, clinical uses, safety, and dietary supplements." *Nutrients.* 14(19): 3934.

59 Nogueira, L.F.R., et al. (2021). "Timing and composition of last meal before bedtime affects sleep parameters of night workers." *Clocks Sleep.* 3(4): 536–46.

60 St-Onge, M.P., et al. (2016). "Effects of diet on sleep quality." *Adv. Nutr.* 7(5): 938–49.

61 Charest, J. and Grandner, M.A. (2020). "Sleep and athletic performance: Impacts on physical performance, mental performance, injury risk and recovery, and mental health." *Sleep Med. Clin.* 15(1): 41–57.

62 Mertens, I.L. and van, Gaal, L.F. (2000). "Overweight, obesity, and blood pressure: The effects of modest weight reduction." *Obesity Research.* 8: 270–78.

63 Yekeen, L.A., et al. (2003). "Prevalence of obesity and high level of cholesterol in hypertension." *Afr J. Biomed Res.* 6: 129–132.

64 Qi, L. et al. (2008). "The common obesity variant near MC4R gene is associated with higher intakes of total energy and dietary fat, weight change and diabetes risk in women." *Human Molecular Genetics.* 17(22): 3502–8.

65 Wolin, K.Y., Carson, K. and Colditz, G.A. (2010). "Obesity and cancer." *The Oncologist.* 15: 556–65.

66 Suk, S–H., et al. (2003). "Abdominal obesity and risk of ischemic stroke: The northern Manhattan stroke study." *Stroke.* 23: 1586–92.

67 Marks, R. (2007). "Obesity profiles with knee osteoarthritis: Correlation with pain, disability, disease progression." *Obesity.* 15: 1867–74.

68 Anderson, K. and Hamm, R.L. (2012). "Factors that impair wound healing." *Journal of the American College of Clinical Wound Specialists.* 4(4): 84–91.

69 Malik, V.S., et al. (2010). "Sugar-sweetened beverages, obesity, type 2 diabetes mellitus, and cardiovascular disease risk." *Circulation.* 121: 1356–64.

70 Anderson, K. and Hamm, R.L. (2012). "Factors that impair wound healing." *Journal of the American College of Clinical Wound Specialists.* 4(4): 84–91.

71 Grover, Steven A., et al. (2015). "Years of life lost and healthy life-years lost from diabetes and cardiovascular disease in overweight and obese people: a modelling study." *The Lancet Diabetes & Endocrinology.* 3(2): 114–22.

72 Poehlman, E.T., et al. (1993). "Determinants of decline in resting metabolic rate in aging females." *AJP-Endocrinology and Metabolism.* 264: 3, E450–E455.

73 Helge, J.W. (2000). "Adaptation to a Fat-Rich Diet." *Sports Med.* 30: 347–57.

74 Gov.uk (2017). "Behind the headlines: calorie guidelines remain unchanged." www.gov.uk/government/news/behind-the-headlines-calorie-guidelines-remain-unchanged [Accessed 8 June 2024]

75   Passmore, R. (1956). "Daily energy expenditure by man." *Proceedings of the Nutrition Society*. 15(1): 83–9.

76   De Souza, R.J., et al. (2015). "Intake of saturated and trans unsaturated fatty acids and risk of all cause mortality, cardiovascular disease, and type 2 diabetes: systematic review and meta-analysis of observational studies." *BMJ*. 351: h3978.

77   Fernandes, A.C., et al. (2019). "Perspective: public health nutrition policies should focus on healthy eating, not on calorie counting, even to decrease obesity." *Adv. Nutr.* 10(4): 549–56.

78   Snow, J.T. and Harris, M.B. (1995). "Maintenance of weight loss after a very-low-calorie diet involving behavioral treatment." *Psychol. Rep.* 76(1): 82.

79   Gardner, C.D., et al. (2022). "Effect of a ketogenic diet versus Mediterranean diet on glycated hemoglobin in individuals with prediabetes and type 2 diabetes mellitus: The interventional Keto-Med randomized crossover trial." *Am. J. Clin. Nutr.* 116(3): 640–52.

80   Juul, F., et al. (2021). "Ultra-processed foods and cardiovascular diseases: Potential mechanisms of action." *Adv. Nutr.* 12(5): 1673–80.

81   Srour, B., et al. (2019). "Ultra-processed food intake and risk of cardiovascular disease: prospective cohort study (NutriNet-Santé)." *BMJ*. 365: l1451.

82   Office for Health Improvements and Disparities (2016). "The Eatwell Guide." www.gov.uk/government/publications/the-eatwell-guide [Accessed 21 May 2024]

83   Katiyar, S.K. and Mukhtar, H. (1997). "Tea antioxidants in cancer chemoprevention." *J. Cell Biochem.* 67: 59–67.

84   Imran, A., et al. (2018). "Exploring the potential of black tea based flavonoids against hyperlipidemia related disorders." *Lipids Health Dis.* 17(1): 57.

85   Fujita, H. and Yamagami, T. (2008). "Antihypercholesterolemic effect of Chinese black tea extract in human subjects with borderline hypercholesterolemia." *Nutr. Res.* 28(7): 450–6.

86   Larsson, S.C., et al. (2013). "Black tea consumption and risk of stroke in women and men." *Ann. Epidemiol.* 23(3): 157–60.

87   Arab, L., et al. (2009). "Green and black tea consumption and risk of stroke: a meta-analysis." *Stroke*. 40(5): 1786–92.

88   Maia, L. and de Mendonça, A. (2002). "Does caffeine intake protect from Alzheimer's disease?" *Eur. J. Neurol.* 9(4): 377–82.

89   Vercambre, M.N., et al. (2013). "Caffeine and cognitive decline in elderly women at high vascular risk." *J. Alzheimers Dis.* 35(2): 413–21.

90   Hedström, A.K., et al. (2016). "High consumption of coffee is associated with decreased multiple sclerosis risk; results from two independent studies." *JNNP*. 87: 454–60.

91   Naveed, M., et al. (2018). "Chlorogenic acid (CGA): A pharmacological review and call for further research." *Biomed. Pharmacother.* 97: 67–74.

92   Schmit, S. L. (2016). "Coffee consumption and the risk of colorectal cancer." *Gruber Cancer Epidemiol Biomarkers Prev.* 25(4): 634–9.

93   Park, S., et al. (2017). "Association of coffee consumption with total and cause-specific mortality among nonwhite populations." *Ann. Intern. Med.* 167: 228–35.

94   Bassett, D.R. Jr., et al. (2017). "Stepc: A review of measurement considerations and health-related applications." *Sports Med.* 47(7): 1303–15.

95   Bennett, G.G., et al. (2006). "Pedometer-determined physical activity among multiethnic low-income housing residents." *Med. Sci. Sports Exerc.* 38(4): 768–73.

96   Mosley. M. (2018). "Forget walking 10,000 steps a day." www.bbc.co.uk/news/health-42864061 [Accessed 21 May 2024]

97   Ohori T., et al. (2012). "Effect of repeated sauna treatment on exercise tolerance and endothelial

function in patients with chronic heart failure." *Am. J. Card.* 109(1): 100–4.

98 Beever R. (2010). "The effects of repeated thermal therapy on quality of life in patients with type II diabetes mellitus." *J. Altern Complement Med.* 16(6): 677–81.

99 Shinsato T., et al. (2010). "Waon therapy mobilizes CD34+ cells and improves peripheral arterial disease." *Journal of Cardiology.* 56(3): 361–6.

100 McCarty, M.F., et al. (2009). "Regular thermal therapy may promote insulin sensitivity while boosting expression of endothelial nitric oxide synthase—Effects comparable to those of exercise training." *Medical Hypotheses.* 73(1): 103–105.

101 Laukkanen T., et al. (2016). "Sauna bathing is inversely associated with dementia and Alzheimer's disease in middle-aged Finnish men." *Age and Ageing.* 46(2): 245–9.

102 Laukkanen T., et al. (2015). "Association between sauna bathing and fatal cardiovascular and all-cause mortality events." *JAMA Internal Medicine.* 175(4): 542–8.

103 Kihara T., et al. (2009). "Waon therapy improves the prognosis of patients with chronic heart failure." *Journal of Cardiology.* 53(2): 214–18.

104 Matsumoto S., et al. (2011). "Effects of thermal therapy combining sauna therapy and underwater exercise in patients with fibromyalgia." *Complementary Therapies in Clinical Practice.* 17(3): 162–6.

105 Oosterveld F. G. J., et al. (2009). "Infrared sauna in patients with rheumatoid arthritis and ankylosing spondylitis." *Clinical Rheumatology.* 28(1): 29–34.

106 Kukkonen-Harjula, K. and Kyllikki Kauppinen, K. (2006). "Health effects and risks of sauna bathing." *Int J. Circumpolar Health.* 65(3): 195–205.

107 Maroon, J.C. and Bost, J.W. (2006). "ω-3 Fatty acids (fish oil) as an anti–inflammatory: an alternative to nonsteroidal anti-inflammatory drugs for discogenic pain." *Surgical Neurology.* 65(4): 326–31.

108 Opperman, M., et al. (2011). "Analysis of omega-3 fatty acid content of South African fish oil supplements." *Cardiovasc J. Afr.* 22(6): 324–9.

109 The Association of UK Dieticians (2021). "Where do Omega-3 fats come from?" https://www.bda.uk.com/resource/omega-3.html [Accessed 21 May 2024]

110 Crupi, R. and Cuzzocrea, S. (2022). "Role of EPA in inflammation: Mechanisms, effects, and clinical relevance." *Biomolecules.* 12(2): 242.

111 Lauritzen, L., et al. (2016). "DHA effects in brain development and function." *Nutrients.* 8(1): 6.

112 Bleakley, C.M. and Davison, G.W. (2010). "Cryotherapy and inflammation: evidence beyond the cardinal signs." *Physical Therapy Reviews.* 15(6): 430–5.

113 Ernst, E. and Fialka, V. (1994). "Ice freezes pain? A review of the clinical effectiveness of analgesic cold therapy." *JPSM.* 9(1): 56–9.

114 Shephard, R.J. (1992). "Fat metabolism, exercise, and the cold." *Canadian Journal of Sport Sciences.* 17(2): 83–90.

115 Giemza, C., et al. (2014). "Effect of cryotherapy on the lumbar spine in elderly men with back pain." *Aging Male.* 17(3): 183–8.

116 Nugraha, B., et al. (2015). "Effects of whole body cryo-chamber therapy on pain in patients with chronic low back pain: A prospective double blind randomised controlled trial." *Eur. J. Phys. Rehabil. Med.* 51: 143–8.

117 Aeberli, I., et al. (2011). "Low to moderate sugar-sweetened beverage consumption impairs glucose and lipid metabolism and promotes inflammation in healthy young men: a randomized controlled trial." *AJCN.* 94(2): 479–85.

118 Nevin, K.G. and Rajamohan, T. (2004). "Beneficial effects of virgin coconut oil on lipid parameters and in vitro LDL oxidation." *Clinical Biochemistry.* 37(9): 830–5.

119 Lacerda Pires Soares, F., et al. (2013). "Gluten-free diet reduces adiposity, inflammation and insulin resistance associated with the induction of PPAR–alpha and PPAR–gamma expression." *JNB*. 24(6): 1105–11.

120 Shaik-Dasthagirisaheb, Y.B., et al. (2013). "Role of vitamins D, E and C in immunity and inflammation." *JBRHA*. 27(2): 291–5.

121 Korntner, S., et al. (2017). "A high-glucose diet affects Achilles tendon healing in rats." *Sci. Rep*. 7: 780.

122 Alcaide-Ruggiero, L., et al. (2021). "Main and minor types of collagens in the articular cartilage: The role of collagens in repair tissue evaluation in chondral defects." *Int. J. Mol. Sci*. 22(24): 13329.

123 De Miranda, R.B., et al. (2021). "Effects of hydrolyzed collagen supplementation on skin aging: a systematic review and meta-analysis." *Int. J. Dermatol*. 60(12): 1449–61.

124 García-Coronado, J.M., et al. (2019). "Effect of collagen supplementation on osteoarthritis symptoms: a meta-analysis of randomized placebo-controlled trials." *Int. Orthop*. 43(3): 531–8.

125 Khatri, M., et al. (2021). "The effects of collagen peptide supplementation on body composition, collagen synthesis, and recovery from joint injury and exercise: A systematic review." *Amino Acids*. 53(10): 1493–506.

126 Hunter, G.R., et al. (2004). "Effects of resistance training on older adults." *Sports Med*. 34(5): 329–48.

127 Schoenfeld, B.J., et al. (2019). "How many times per week should a muscle be trained to maximize muscle hypertrophy? A systematic review and meta-analysis of studies examining the effects of resistance training frequency." *J. Sports Sci*. 37(11): 1286–95.

128 Borde, R., et al. (2015). "Dose-response relationships of resistance training in healthy old adults: A systematic review and meta-analysis." *Sports Med*. 45(12): 1693–720.

129 Iraki, J., et al. (2019). "Nutrition recommendations for bodybuilders in the off-season: A narrative review." *Sports (Basel)*. 7(7): 154.

130 Aoki, K.C. and Mayrovitz, H.N. (2022). "Utility of a body shape index parameter in predicting cardiovascular disease risks." *Cureus*. 14(4): e23886.

131 Martin, C.K., et al. (2022). CALERIE™ Phase 2 Study Group. "Challenges in defining successful adherence to calorie restriction goals in humans: Results from CALERIE™ 2." *Exp Gerontol*. 162: 111757.

132 Dinan, T.G., et al. (2015). "Collective unconscious: how gut microbes shape human behavior." *J. Psychiatr. Res*. 63: 1–9.

133 Calbet, J.A.L., et al. (2017). "Exercise preserves lean mass and performance during severe energy deficit: The role of exercise volume and dietary protein content." *Front. Physiol*. 8: 483.

134 Duregon, E., et al. (2021). "Intermittent fasting: from calories to time restriction." *Geroscience*. 43(3): 1083–92.

135 Tian, Y., et al.(2013). "Exploring the system-wides costs of falls in older people in Torbay." https://www.kingsfund.org.uk/insight-and-analysis/reports/system-wide-costs-falls-older-people-torbay [Accessed 21 May 2024]

136 Guzon-Illescas, O., et al. (2019). "Mortality after osteoporotic hip fracture: incidence, trends, and associated factors." *J. Orthop. Surg. Res*. 14(1): 203.

137 Nishikawa, K.C., et al. (2018). "Basic science and clinical use of eccentric contractions: History and uncertainties." *J. Sport Health Sci*. 7(3): 265–74.

138 Volpi, E., et al. (2004). "Muscle tissue changes with aging." *Curr. Opin. Clin. Nutr. Metab. Care*. 7(4): 405–10.

139 Hsieh, H.F. and Lee, F.P. (2005). "Graduated compression stockings as prophylaxis for flight-related venous thrombosis: systematic literature review." *J. Adv. Nurs*. 51(1): 83–98.

Part Eight: The Power of the Mind

1   Brinjikji, W., et al. (2015). "Systematic literature review of imaging features of spinal degeneration in asymptomatic populations." *AJNR Am. J. Neuroradiol.* 36(4): 811–16.

2   Negendank, W.G., et al. (1990). "Magnetic resonance imaging of meniscal degeneration in asymptomatic knees." *J. Orthop Res.* 8: 311–20.

3   Okada, E., et al. (2011). "Disc degeneration of cervical spine on MRI in patients with lumbar disc herniation: comparison study with asymptomatic volunteers." *Eur. Spine J.* 20: 585.

4   Puentedura, E.J. and Leuw, A. (2012). "A neuroscience approach to managing athletes with low back pain." *Physical Therapy in Sport.* 13: 123–33.

5   TedX Adelaide—Lorimer Mosely (2011). "Why things hurt." https://www.youtube.com/watch?v=gwd-wLdIHjs [Accessed 21 May 2024]

6   Nestor, J. (2021). *Breath: The new science of a lost art.* London: Penguin.

7   Owoeye, O.B.A., et al. (2022). "Absence of injury is not absence of pain: Prevalence of preseason musculoskeletal pain and associated factors in collegiate soccer and basketball student athletes." *Int. J. Environ. Res. Public Health.* 19 (15): 9128.

8   Hawkins, S.A., et al. (2001). "Low-involvement learning: Repetition and coherence in familiarity and belief." *Journal of Consumer Psychology.* 11(1): 1–11.

9   Majeed, M.H., et al. (2018). "Mindfulness based interventions for chronic pain: evidence and application." *Asian Journal of Psychiatry.* 32: 79–82.

10 Tavallaei, V., et al. (2018). "Mindfulness for female outpatients with chronic primary headaches: an internet-based bibliotherapy." *Eur. J. Transl. Myol.* 28(2): 175–84.

11 Cohen, S., et al. (2012). "Stress, GCR, inflammation, and disease risk." *Proceedings of the National Academy of Sciences.* 109(16): 5995–9.

12 Sapse, A.T. (1984). "Stress, cortisol, interferon and 'stress' diseases: I. Cortisol as the cause of 'stress' diseases." *Medical Hypotheses.* 13(1): 31–44.

13 Saul, A.N., et al. (2005). "Chronic stress and susceptibility to skin cancer." *JNCI.* 97(23): 1760–7.

14 Robles, T. F., et al. (2005). "Out of balance: A new look at chronic stress, depression, and immunity." *Current Directions in Psychological Science,* 14(2): 111–15.

15 Teut, M., et al. (2013). "Mindful walking in psychologically distressed individuals: a randomized controlled trial." *Evid. Based Complement Alternat. Med.* 2013: 489856.

16 Jin, P. (1992). "Efficacy of Tai Chi, brisk walking, meditation, and reading in reducing mental and emotional stress." *J. Psychosom. Res.* 36(4): 361–70.

17 Russell, D., et al. (1984). "Social and emotional loneliness: An examination of Weiss's typology of loneliness." *J. Pers Soc Psychol.* 46(6): 1313–21.

18 Ledford, A.K., et al. (2022). "Psychological and physiological changes during basic, underwater, demolition/SEAL training." *Physiol. Behav.* 257: 113970.

19 Keller, A., et al. (2012). "Does the perception that stress affects health matter? The association with health and mortality." *Health Psychol.* 31(5): 677–84.

20 Costigan, M., et al. (2009). "Neuropathic pain: A maladaptive response of the nervous system to damage." *Annu. Rev. Neurosci.* 32: 1–32.

21 Goldstein, P., et al. (2017). "The role of touch in regulating inter-partner physiological coupling during empathy for pain." *Sci. Rep.* 7(1): 3252.

22 Testa, M. and Rossettini G. (2016). "Enhance placebo, avoid nocebo: How contextual factors affect physiotherapy outcomes." *Man. Ther.* 24: 65–74.

23 Ji, R.R., et al. (2018). "Neuroinflammation and central sensitization in chronic and widespread pain." *Anesthesiology*. 129(2): 343–66.

24 Birke, H., et al. (2019). "Chronic pain, opioid therapy, sexual desire, and satisfaction in sexual life: A population-based survey." *Pain Med*. 20(6): 1132–40.

25 Matsuura, T., et al. (2016). "Relationship between oxytocin and pain modulation and inflammation." *J. UOEH*. 38(4): 325–34.

26 Sidorkewicz, N. and McGill, S.M. (2015). "Documenting female spine motion during coitus with a commentary on the implications for the low back pain patient." *Eur. Spine J*. 24(3): 513–20.

27 Sidorkewicz, N. and McGill, S.M. (2014). "Male spine motion during coitus: implications for the low back pain patient." *Spine* (Phila. Pa. 1976). 39(20): 1633–9.

28 Chen, L.F., et al. (2015). "The Hawthorne effect in infection prevention and epidemiology." *Infect. Control. Hosp. Epidemiol*. 36(12): 1444–50.

29 Ferriss, T. (2017). "Fear-setting: The most valuable exercise I do every month." https://tim.blog/2017/05/15/fear-setting/ [Accessed 21 May 2024]

30 Hanning, U., et al. (2016). "Structural brain changes and all-cause mortality in the elderly population—the mediating role of inflammation." *Age* (Dordr). 38(5–6): 455–64.

31 World Health Organization (2023). "Mental health of older adults." www.who.int/news-room/fact-sheets/detail/mental-health-of-older-adults [Accessed 21 May 2024]

32 Erzen, E. and Çikrikci, Ö. (2018). "The effect of loneliness on depression: A meta-analysis." *Int. J. Soc. Psychiatry*. 64(5): 427–35.

33 Staff, R. (2018). "Regular problem solving does not protect against mental decline." https://www.abdn.ac.uk/news/12537/ [Accessed 21 May 2024]

34 Fu, C., et al. (2018). "Association between social activities and cognitive function among the elderly in China: A cross-sectional study." *Int. J. Environ. Res. Public Health*. 15(2): 231.

35 Bernardo, T.C., et al. (2016). "Physical exercise and brain mitochondrial fitness: The possible role against Alzheimer's disease." *Brain Pathol*. 26(5): 648–63.

36 Khazaee-Pool, M., et al. (2015). "Effects of physical exercise programme on happiness among older people." *J. Psychiatr. Ment. Health Nurs*. 22(1): 47–57.

37 Son, W.M., et al. (2017). "Combined exercise reduces arterial stiffness, blood pressure, and blood markers for cardiovascular risk in postmenopausal women with hypertension." *Menopause*. 24(3): 262–8.

38 Kuiper J.S., et al. (2015). "Social relationships and risk of dementia: A systematic review and meta–analysis of longitudinal cohort studies." *Ageing Res. Rev*. 22: 39–57.

39 Zhong, G., et al. (2015). "Smoking is associated with an increased risk of dementia: a meta-analysis of prospective cohort studies with investigation of potential effect modifiers." *PLoS One*. 10(3): e0118333.

40 University of Exeter (2014). "Why plants in the office make us more productive." www.exeter.ac.uk/news/featurednews/title_409094_en.html [Accessed 21 May 2024]

41 Bang, K.S., et al. (2017). "The effects of a campus forest-walking program on undergraduate and graduate students' physical and psychological health." *Int. J. Environ. Res. Public Health*. 14(7): ii, E728.

42 Alquist, J. and Baumeister, R.F. (2012). "Self-control: limited resources and extensive benefits." *Wiley Interdiscip Rev Cogn Sci*. 3(3): 419–23.

43 Cox, D. (2017). "Pain is the body's way of telling us to be careful—but there are some who go their entire lives without feeling it. Could their disorder unlock new ways to safely deal with chronic pain?" www.bbc.com/future/article/20170426-the-people-who-never-feel-any-pain [Accessed 21 May 2024]

Resources

The videos mentioned in the book can be accessed via my website: **ht-physio.co.uk**.

- Video A: Back Pain Relief through Breathing

- Video B: The Tiny Muscle Responsible for a Lot of Back Trouble

- Video C: A Simple Trick for Sciatica Calf Pain Relief

- Video D: What to Do When Knee Pain Affects Your Walking

- Video E: Reconnect with Your Feet

- Video F: The Problem with Tight Calves

- Video G: How to Get Up from the Floor #1

- Video H: How to Get Up from the Floor #2

- Video I: 12 Tips to Fix Your Walking

I hope you'll consider downloading my free gift to you with this book: "The Top 5 Exercises for Over-50s Who Want to Remain Strong, Mobile & Active." I've laid out the benefits of resistance training on page 288, and this free downloadable guide will show you the way to achieve those benefits in later life. It is quite literally a roadmap to achieving strength, mobility and health. It just needs a little effort on your part, but I know you'll be able to get there. You can find this valuable guide and take it for free at: **ht-physio.co.uk/guide/**.

If you've enjoyed this book, you'll find hundreds of bite-sized lessons, demonstrations and exercises on our YouTube channel: **YouTube.com/@HT-physio**.

Be sure to subscribe to the channel and leave a comment letting us know you have read the book!

If you are in the Farnham, Surrey area, why not get in touch to ask us how we can help you to recover from a painful problem? You can find all the contact details you'll need at my website.

If you are serious about improving your strength, mobility, balance and independence, there is no better way to do this than to join my Lifelong Mobility™ program. Inside this special members' area, you'll find my best exercise routines (which you can follow along with at home) and other content to help you improve your health that can't be found anywhere else. You can learn more about Lifelong Mobility™ at **willharlow. com/lifelong**.

Index

Exercises are in *italics*

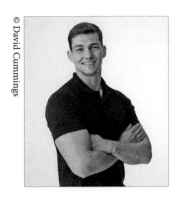

© David Cummings

About the Author

Will Harlow is a physiotherapist with a mission to help over-fifties stay mobile, healthy and active, without the use of pain pills or surgery.

He graduated from Brunel University in 2015, where he received a first-class master's degree in physiotherapy. He then went on to work in the NHS as a junior, senior and team leader. He also enjoyed a stint working in professional football for the biggest football club on the south coast of England.

He now works and lives in Surrey, running his private physiotherapy practice, HT Physio, in Farnham.

In his spare time, Will enjoys the gym, travel and collecting funk, soul and disco records. He lives with his wife, Bryony, and their cat, Zeus.

🌐 ht-physio.co.uk

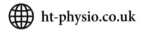 @HT-Physio

𝐟 @HTPhysioUK

📷 @HTPhysioOfficial

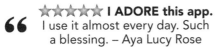

CONNECT WITH
HAY HOUSE
ONLINE

🌐 hayhouse.co.uk   **f** @hayhouse

📷 @hayhouseuk   𝕏 @hayhouseuk

▶️ @hayhouseuk   ♪ @hayhouseuk

Find out all about our latest books & card decks • Be the first to know about exclusive discounts • Interact with our authors in live broadcasts • Celebrate the cycle of the seasons with us • Watch free videos from your favourite authors • Connect with like-minded souls

'The gateways to wisdom and knowledge are always open.'

Louise Hay